The RENAL Diet COOKBOOK

The Complete Ultimate Guide To Discover Delicious, Healthy, Low Sodium, Low Potassium & Phosphorus Kidney Receipts for Easy Meal Ideas to Managing CKD and Avoiding Dialysis

Glenda Hamilton

Table of Contents

CHAPTER 6 - SEAFOOD RECIPES 59

CHAPTER 7 - POULTRY AND MEAT RECIPES 73

CHAPTER 8 - SALAD RECIPES 87

CHAPTER 9 - DESSERT RECIPES 99

INTRODUCTION

Human **health hangs in a** complete balance when all of its interconnected bodily mechanisms function properly in perfect sync. Without its major organs working normally, the body soon suffers indelible damage. Kidney malfunction is one such example, and it is not just the entire water balance that is disturbed by kidney disease, but some other ailments also emerge due to this problem.

However, all forms of renal diet have one thing in common, which is to improve your renal functions, bring some relief to your kidneys, as well as prevent kidneys disease at patients with numerous risk factors, altogether improving your overall health and well-being. The grocery list we have provided should help you get ahold of which groceries you should introduce to your diet and which groups of food should be avoided in order to improve your kidneys' performance, so you can start from shopping for your new lifestyle.

You don't need to shop many different types of groceries all at once as it is always better to use fresh produce, although frozen food also makes a good alternative when fresh fruit and vegetables are not available.

As far as the renal diet we are recommending in our guide, this form of kidney-friendly dietary regimen offers solution in form of low-sodium and low-potassium meals and groceries, which is why we are also offering simple and easy renal diet recipes in our guide. By following a dietary plan compiled for all stages of renal system failure unless the doctor recommends a different treatment by allowing or expelling some of the groceries, we have listed in our ultimate grocery list for renal patients.

Before we get to cooking and changing your lifestyle from the very core with the idea of improving your health, we want you to get familiar with renal diet basics and find out exactly what this diet is based on while you already know what is the very core solution found in renal diet – helping you improve your kidney's health by lowering sodium and potassium intake.

Despite their tiny size, the kidneys perform several functions which are vital for the body to be able to function healthily.

These functions include:

1. Filtering redundant fluids and waste from the blood.
2. Creating the enzyme known as renin that regulates the blood pressure.
3. Ensuring bone marrow creates red blood cells.
4. Controlling calcium and phosphorus levels through absorption and excretion.

Unfortunately, when kidney disease reaches a chronic stage, these functions begin to fail. However, with the right treatment and lifestyle, it is possible to manage symptoms and continue living well. This is even more applicable in the earlier stages of the disease. Tactlessly, 10% of all adults over the age of 20 will experience some form of kidney disease in their lifetime. Depend on the cause, a variety of different treatments for kidney disease can be found.

Kidney (or renal) diseases are affecting around 14% of the adult population according to international stats. In the US, approx. 661.000 Americans suffer from kidney dysfunction. Out of these patients, 468.000 proceed to dialysis treatment and the rest have one active kidney transplant.

The high quantities of diabetes and heart illness are additionally related to kidney dysfunction and sometimes one condition, for example, diabetes may prompt the other.

With such a significant number of high rates, possibly the best course of treatment is the contravention of dialysis, which makes people depend upon clinical and crisis facility meds on any occasion multiple times every week. In this way, if your kidney has just given a few indications of malfunctioning, you can forestall dialysis through an eating routine, something that we will talk about in this book.

CHAPTER 1 - UNDERSTANDING KIDNEY DISEASE

Kidney disease is becoming more prevalent in the United States; therefore, we need to learn as much about it as we can. Once you understand what chronic kidney disease is, you can begin to take charge of your evolving health needs. Making healthy changes early in the stages of this ailment will help determine how well you will manage your kidney health. Like any new process, it may seem intimidating at first. But this provides the foundation for learning and will help you understand the illness as you begin your journey to healthier kidneys.

1.1   How Do the Kidneys Work?

Our kidneys are small but they do powerful things to keep our bodies in balance. They are bean-shaped, about the size of a fist, and are located in the middle of the back, on the left and right sides of the spine, just below the rib cage. When everything is working properly, the kidneys do many important jobs such as:

5.   Filter waste materials from the blood.
6.   Remove extra fluid, or water, from the body.
7.   Release hormones that help manage blood pressure.
8.   Stimulate bone marrow to make red blood cells.

1.2   What Causes Kidney Disease?

So many things cause kidney disease, including damage because of physical injury or disorders, but the 2 leading causes are diabetes and high blood pressure. These underlying conditions also put people at risk for developing cardiovascular disease. Early treatment may not only slow down the progression of the illness, but also reduce your risk of developing heart disease or stroke.

African Americans, Hispanics, and American Indians are at increased risk for kidney failure because these groups have a greater prevalence of diabetes and high blood pressure.

When we digest protein, our bodies create waste products. As blood flows through the capillaries, the waste products are filtered through the urine. Substances such as protein and red blood cells are too big to pass through the capillaries, and so, stay in the blood. All the extra work takes a toll on the kidneys. When kidney disease is detected in the early stages, several treatments may prevent the worsening of the disease. If it is detected in the later stages, high amounts of protein in your urine, called macroalbuminuria, can lead to end-stage renal disease.

The second leading cause of kidney disease is high blood pressure, also known as hypertension. Although there is no cure for hypertension, certain medications, a low-sodium diet, and physical activity can lower blood pressure.

The kidneys help manage blood pressure, but when it is high, the heart has to work overtime at pumping blood. When the force of blood flow is elevated, blood vessels start to stretch so the blood can flow more easily. The stretching and scarring weaken the blood vessels throughout the entire body, including the kidneys. And when the kidneys' blood vessels are injured, they may not remove the waste and extra fluid from the body, creating a dangerous cycle, because the extra fluid in the blood vessels can increase blood pressure even more.

With diabetes, excess blood sugar remains in the bloodstream. The high blood sugar levels can damage the blood vessels in the kidneys and elsewhere in the body. And since high blood pressure is a complication from diabetes, the extra pressure can make the walls of the blood vessels week, which can lead to a heart attack or stroke.

Other conditions, such as drug abuse and certain autoimmune diseases, can also cause injury to the kidneys. In fact, every drug we put into our body has to pass through the kidneys for filtration.

An autoimmune disease means the immune system, which is designed to protect the body from illness, sees the body as an invader and attacks its own systems, including the kidneys. Some forms of lupus, for example, attack the kidneys. Another autoimmune disease that can lead to kidney failure is Goodpasture syndrome, a group of conditions that affect the kidneys and the lungs. The damage to the kidneys from autoimmune diseases can lead to chronic kidney disease and kidney failure.

1.3 Symptoms of Kidney Disease

The good thing is that we can prevent the chronic stage of renal disease by identifying the early signs of any form of kidney damage. Even when a person feels minor changes in his body, they should consult an expert to confirm if it might lead to something serious. The following are a few of the early symptoms of renal damage:

- Tiredness or drowsiness
- Muscle cramps
- Loss of appetite
- Changes in the frequency of urination
- Swelling of hands and feet
- A feeling of itchiness

- Numbness
- The darkness of skin
- Trouble in sleeping

- Shortness of breath
- The feeling of nausea or vomiting

These symptoms can appear in combination with one another. These are general signs of body malfunction, and they should never be ignored. And if they are left unnoticed, they can lead to worsening of the condition and may appear as:

- Back pain
- Abdominal pain
- Fever
- Rash

- Diarrhea
- Nosebleeds
- Vomiting

After witnessing any of these symptoms, a person should immediately consult a health expert and prepare themself for the required lifestyle changes.

1.4   Stages of Kidney Disease

According to the National Kidney Foundation in the US, kidney disease can be classified into 5 different progressive stages. These stages and their symptoms do not only help the doctor to devise an appropriate therapy, but also guide the patient to take the necessary measures in routine life. The rate of kidney function actually talks much about these phases. In the early stages, there is minimum loss of function, and this loss increases with every stage.

The eGFR is used as a standard criterion to measure kidney function. eGFR is the acronym for the estimated Glomerular Filtration Rate. It is the rate at which the waste material is transferred from the blood to the nephron's tubes through the "glomerulus"—the filtering membrane of the kidney tissues. The lesser the rate of glomerular filtration, the greater the problem the kidneys are going through. A person's age, gender, race, and serum creatinine are entered into a mathematical formula to calculate their eGFR. The serum creatinine level is measured in a blood test. Creatinine is actually a waste product of the body which is produced out of muscular activities. Healthy kidneys are capable of removing all the creatinine out of the blood. A rising creatinine level is, therefore, a sign of kidney disease. It is said that if a person has been having an eGFR of less than 60 for 3 months, it means that they are suffering from serious renal problems.

The 5 main stages of chronic kidney disease can be categorized as follows:

9. Stage 1: The first stage starts when the eGFR gets slightly higher than the normal value. In this stage, the eGFR can be equal to or greater than 90mL/min.
10. Stage 2: The next stage arises when the eGFR starts to decline and ranges between 60–89 mL/min. It is best to control the progression of the disease at this point.
11. Stage 3: From this point on, kidney disease becomes concerning for the patient as the eGFR drops to 30–59 mL/min. At this stage, consultation is essential for the health of the patient.
12. Stage 4: Stage 4 is also known as Severe Chronic Kidney Disease as the eGFR level drops to 15–29 mL/min.
13. Stage 5: The final and most critical phase of chronic renal disease is stage 5, where the estimated glomerular filtration rate gets as low as below 15 mL/min.

1.5   Renal Disease Diagnostic Tests

Besides identifying the symptoms of kidney disease, there are other better and more accurate ways to confirm the extent of loss of renal function. There are mainly 2 important diagnostic tests:

1. Urine test: The urine test clearly states all the renal problems. The urine is the waste product of the kidney. When there is a loss of filtration or any hindrance to the kidneys, the urine sample will indicate it through the number of excretory products present in it. The severe stages of chronic disease show some amount of protein and blood in the urine. Do not rely on self-tests; visit an authentic clinic for these tests.

2. Blood pressure and blood test: Another good way to check for renal disease is to test the blood and its composition. A high amount of creatinine and other waste products in the blood clearly indicates that the kidneys are not functioning properly. Blood pressure can also be indicative of renal disease. When the water balance in the body is disturbed, it may cause high blood pressure. Hypertension can both be the cause and symptom of kidney disease, and therefore, should be taken seriously.

1.6   Treatment Plans for Chronic Kidney Disease (CKD)

The best way to manage CKD is to be an active participant in your treatment program, regardless of your stage of renal disease. Proper treatment involves a combination of working with a healthcare team, adhering to a renal diet, and making healthy lifestyle decisions. These can all have a profoundly positive effect on your kidney disease—especially watching how you eat.

3. Working with your healthcare team. When you have kidney disease, working in partnership with your healthcare team can be extremely important in your treatment program as well as being personally empowering. Regularly meeting with your physician or healthcare team can arm you with resources, and provide you with a much-needed opportunity to vent, share information, get advice, and receive support in effectively managing this illness.

4. Adhering to a renal diet. The heart of this book is the renal diet. Sticking to this diet can make a huge difference in your health and vitality. Like any change, following the diet may not be easy at first. Important changes to your diet, particularly early on, can possibly prevent the need for dialysis. These changes include limiting salt, eating a low-protein diet, reducing fat intake, and getting enough calories if you need to lose weight. Be honest with yourself first and foremost—learn what you need, and consider your personal goals and obstacles. Start by making small changes. It is okay to have some slip-ups—we all do. With guidance and support, these small changes will become habits of your promising new lifestyle. In no time, you will begin taking control of your diet and health.

5. Making healthy lifestyle decisions. Lifestyle choices play a crucial part in our health, especially when it comes to helping regulate kidney disease. Lifestyle choices such as allotting time for physical activity, getting enough sleep, managing weight, reducing stress, and limiting smoking and alcohol will help you take control of your overall health, making it easier to manage your kidney disease. Follow this simple formula: Keep toxins out of your body as much as you can and build up your immune system with a good balance of exercise, relaxation, and sleep.

CHAPTER 2 - TYPES OF FOOD YOU CAN EAT

The renal diet aims to cut down the amount of waste in the blood. When people have kidney dysfunction, the kidneys are unable to remove and filter waste properly. When waste is left in the blood, it can affect the electrolyte levels of the patient. With a kidney diet, kidney function is promoted, and the progression of complete kidney failure is slowed down.

The renal diet follows a low intake of proteins, phosphorus, and sodium. It is necessary to consume high-quality proteins and limit some fluids. For some people, it is important to limit calcium and potassium.

Promoting a renal diet, here are the substances which are critical to be monitored:

2.1   Sodium and Its Role in the Body

Most natural foods contain sodium. Some people think that sodium and salt are interchangeable. However, salt is a compound of chloride and sodium. There might be either salt or sodium in other forms in the food we eat. Due to the added salt, processed foods include a higher level of sodium.

Apart from potassium and chloride, sodium is one of the most crucial body's electrolytes. The main function of electrolytes is to control the fluids when they are going out and in the body's cells and tissues.

With sodium:

- Blood volume and pressure are regulated.

- Muscle contraction and nerve function are regulated.
- The acid-base balance of the blood is regulated.

- The amount of fluid the body eliminates and keeps is balanced.

Why is it important to monitor sodium intake for people with kidney issues?

Since failing kidneys are unable to reduce excess fluid and sodium from the body adequately, too much sodium might be harmful. As fluid and sodium build up in the bloodstream and tissues, they might cause:

- Edema—swelling in face, hands, and legs.
- Increased thirst.
- High blood pressure.

- Shortness of breath.
- Heart failure.

The ways to monitor sodium intake:

- Avoid processed foods.
- Be attentive to serving sizes.
- Read food labels.
- Use fresh meats instead of processed.
- Choose fresh fruits and veggies.

- Compare brands, choosing the ones with the lowest sodium levels.
- Use spices that do not include salt.
- Ensure the sodium content is less than 400 mg. per meal and not more than 150 mg. per snack.
- Cook at home, not adding salt.

Foods to eat with lower sodium content:

6. Fresh meats, dairy products, frozen veggies, and fruits.
7. Fresh herbs and seasonings like rosemary, oregano, dill, lime, cilantro, onion, lemon, and garlic.
8. Corn tortilla chips, pretzels, no salt added crackers, unsalted popcorn.

2.2 Potassium and Its Role in the Body

The main function of potassium is keeping muscles working correctly and the heartbeat regular. This mineral is responsible for maintaining electrolyte and fluid balance in the bloodstream. The kidneys regulate the proper amount of potassium in the body, expelling excess amounts in the urine.

The ways to monitor potassium intake:

- Limit high potassium food.
- Select only fresh fruits and veggies.
- Limit dairy products and milk to 8 oz. per day.

- Avoid potassium chloride.
- Read labels on packaged foods.
- Avoid seasonings and salt substitutes with potassium.

Foods to eat with lower potassium:

9. Fruits: Watermelon, tangerines, pineapple, plums, peaches, pears, papayas, mangoes, lemons and limes, honeydew, grapefruit/grapefruit juice, grapes/grape juice, clementine/satsuma, cranberry juice, berries, and apples/applesauce, apple juice.

10. Veggies: Summer squash (cooked), okra, mushrooms (fresh), lettuce, kale, green beans, eggplant, cucumber, corn, onions (raw), celery, cauliflower, carrots, cabbage, broccoli (fresh), bamboo shoots (canned), and bell peppers.

11. Plain Turkish delights, marshmallows and jellies, boiled fruit sweets, and peppermints.

12. Shortbread, ginger nut biscuits, plain digestives.

13. Plain flapjacks and cereal bars.

14. Plain sponge cakes like Madeira cake, lemon sponge, jam sponge.

15. Corn-based and wheat crisps.

16. Whole grain crispbreads and crackers.

17. Protein and other foods (bread (not whole grain), pasta, noodles, rice, eggs, canned tuna, turkey (white meat), and chicken (white meat).

2.3 Phosphorus and Its Role in the Body

This mineral is essential in bone development and maintenance. Phosphorus helps in the development of connective organs and tissue and assists in muscle movement. Extra phosphorus is possible to be removed by healthy kidneys; however, it is impossible with kidney dysfunction. High levels of phosphorus make bones week by pulling calcium out of your bones. It might lead to dangerous calcium deposits in the heart, eyes, lungs, and blood vessels.

The ways to monitor phosphorus intake:

18. Pay attention to serving size.

19. Eat fresh fruits and veggies.

20. Eat smaller portions of foods that are rich in proteins.

21. Avoid packaged foods.

22. Keep a food journal.

    Foods to eat with lower phosphorus levels:

23. Grapes, apples.

24. Lettuce, leeks.

25. Carbs (white rice, corn, and rice cereal, popcorn, pasta, crackers (not wheat), white bread).

26. Meat (sausage, fresh meat).

2.4 Protein and Its Role in the Body

Damaged kidneys are unable to remove protein waste, so they accumulate in the blood. The amount of protein to consume differs depending on the stage of CKD. Protein is critical for tissue maintenance, and it is necessary to eat the proper amount of it according to the particular stage of kidney disease.

Sources of protein for vegetarians:

27. Vegans (allowing only plant-based foods): Wheat protein and whole grains, nut butter, soy protein, yogurt, or soy milk, cooked no salt added canned and dried beans and peas, unsalted nuts.

28. Lacto vegetarians (allowing dairy products, milk, and plant-based foods): Reduced-sodium or low-sodium cottage cheese.

29. Lacto-ovo vegetarians (allowing eggs, dairy products, milk, and plant-based foods): Eggs.

THE RENAL DIET COOKBOOK

CHAPTER 3 - BREAKFAST RECIPES

3.1   CHEESE SPAGHETTI FRITTATA

Preparation time: 10 minutes - Cooking time: 10 minutes - Servings: 2

Ingredients

4 c. whole wheat spaghetti, cooked

- 4 tsps. olive oil
- 4 large eggs
- ½ c. milk
- ⅓ c. Parmesan cheese, grated
- 2 tbsps. fresh parsley, chopped
- 2 tbsps. fresh basil, chopped
- ½ tsp. black pepper
- 1 tomato, diced

Directions

1. Set a suitable nonstick skillet over moderate heat and add olive oil.
2. Place spaghetti in the skillet and cook by stirring for 2 minutes on moderate heat.
3. Whisk the eggs with milk, parsley, and black pepper in a bowl.
4. Pour this milky egg mixture over the spaghetti and top it all with basil, cheese, and tomato.
5. Cover the spaghetti frittata again with a lid and cook for approximately 8 minutes on low heat.
6. Slice and serve.

Nutrition

- Calories: 230
- Total fat: 7.8 g.
- Sodium: 77 mg.
- Dietary fiber: 5.6 g.
- Sugar: 4.5 g.
- Protein: 11.1 g.
- Calcium: 88 mg.
- Phosphorus: 368 mg.
- Potassium: 214 mg.

3.2   SHRIMP BRUSCHETTA

Preparation time: 15 minutes - Cooking time: 10 minutes - Servings: 4

Ingredients

- 13 oz. shrimps, peeled
- 1 tbsp. tomato sauce
- ½ tsp. Splenda
- ¼ tsp. garlic powder
- 1 tsp. fresh parsley, chopped
- ½ tsp. olive oil
- 1 tsp. lemon juice
- 4 whole grain bread slices
- 1 c. water, for cooking

Directions

1. In the saucepan, pour water and bring it to boil.
2. Add shrimps and boil them over high heat for 5 minutes.
3. After this, drain shrimps and chill them to room temperature.
4. Mix up together shrimps with Splenda, garlic powder, tomato sauce, and fresh parsley.
5. Add lemon juice and stir gently.
6. Preheat the oven to 360°F.
7. Coat the slice of bread with olive oil and bake for 3 minutes.
8. Then place the shrimp mixture on the bread. Bruschetta is cooked.

Nutrition

- Calories: 199
- Fat: 3.7 g.
- Fiber: 2.1 g.
- Carbohydrates: 15.3 g.
- Protein: 24.1 g.
- Calcium: 79 mg.
- Phosphorus: 316 mg.
- Potassium: 227 mg.
- Sodium: 121 mg.

3.3   STRAWBERRY MUESLI

Preparation time: 10 minutes - Cooking time: 30 minutes - Servings: 4

Ingredients

- 2 c. Greek yogurt
- 1 ½ c. strawberries, sliced
- 1 ½ c. Muesli
- 4 tsp. maple syrup
- ¾ tsp. ground cinnamon

Directions

1. Put Greek yogurt in the food processor.
2. Add 1 c. strawberries, maple syrup, and ground cinnamon.
3. Blend the ingredients until you get a smooth mass.
4. Transfer the yogurt mass into the serving bowls.
5. Add Muesli and stir well.

6. Leave the meal for 30 minutes in the fridge.
7. After this, decorate it with the remaining sliced strawberries.

Nutrition

- Calories: 149
- Fat: 2.6 g.
- Fiber: 3.6 g.
- Carbohydrates: 21.6 g.
- Protein: 12 g.

- Calcium: 69 mg.
- Phosphorus: 216 mg.
- Potassium: 227 mg.
- Sodium: 151 mg.

3.4 YOGURT BULGUR

Preparation time: 10 minutes - Cooking time: 15 minutes - Servings: 3

Ingredients

- 1 c. bulgur
- 2 c. Greek yogurt
- 1 ½ c. water

- ½ tsp. salt
- 1 tsp. olive oil

Directions

1. Pour olive oil into the saucepan and add bulgur.
2. Roast it over medium heat for 2–3 minutes. Stir it from time to time.
3. After this, add salt and water.
4. Close the lid and cook bulgur for 15 minutes over medium heat.
5. Then chill the cooked bulgur well and combine it with Greek yogurt. Stir it carefully.
6. Transfer the cooked meal to the serving plates. The yogurt bulgur tastes the best when it is cold.

Nutrition

- Calories: 274
- Fat: 4.9 g.
- Fiber: 8.5 g.
- Carbohydrates: 40.8 g.
7. Sodium: 131 mg.

- Protein: 19.2 g.Calcium: 39 mg.
- Phosphorus: 216 mg.
- Potassium: 237 mg.

3.5   BACON AND CHEESE CRUSTLESS QUICHE

Preparation time: 10 minutes - Cooking time: 4 hours - Servings: 6

Ingredients

- 1 tbsp. butter
- 10 beaten eggs
- 8 oz. shredded Cheddar cheese, reduced-fat
- 1 c. light cream
- ½ tbsp. black pepper
- 10 pieces chopped bacon, cooked

Directions

1. Grease your Slow Cooker with butter and set aside.
2. Combine eggs, cheese, cream, and pepper in a mixing bowl. Add mixture into the Slow Cooker.
3. Splash bacon over the mixture and cover the Slow Cooker.
4. Cook for about 4 hours on low. Make sure the quiche is not over-cooked.
5. Serve and enjoy.

Nutrition

- Calories: 436
- Total fat: 36 g.
- Saturated fat: 16 g.
- Total carbohydrates: 4 g.
- Protein: 24 g.
- Sugar: 1.6 g.
- Fiber: 0.5 g.
- Sodium: 631 mg.
- Potassium: 30.8 g.

3.6   MUSHROOM CRUSTLESS QUICHE

Preparation time: 15 minutes - Cooking time: 4 hours - Servings: 6

Ingredients

- 3 tbsp. butter, divided
- 1 package, 10 oz., sliced mushrooms
- 1 red bell pepper, 1-inch strips
- ¼ tbsp. kosher salt
- 1 tbsp. minced onion, dried
- 10 beaten eggs
- ½ tbsp. black pepper
- 1 c. light cream
- 1 package, 10 oz., shredded Cheddar cheese, reduced-fat

Directions

1. Grease your Slow Cooker with 1 tbsp. butter.
2. Heat 2 tbsp. butter in a skillet for about 30 seconds over medium heat then add mushrooms, peppers, salt, and onions.
3. Sauté for about 5 minutes until mushrooms lose water and pepper softens. Drain vegetables and transfer to the Slow Cooker.
4. Whisk together eggs, black pepper, cream, and cheese in a mixing bowl.
5. Add the egg mixture to vegetables into the Slow Cooker then stir to combine.
6. Cover the Slow Cooker and cook for about 4 hours on low. Make sure it is not to overcook.
7. Serve and enjoy.

Nutrition

- Calories: 429
- Total fat: 35 g.
- Saturated fat: 20 g.
- Total carbohydrates: 5.3 g.
- Protein: 23.2 g.

- Sugar: 2.7 g.
- Fiber: 0.9 g.
- Sodium: 738 mg.
- Potassium: 362 mg.

3.7   MAPLE GLAZED WALNUTS

Preparation time: 15 minutes - Cooking time: 2 hours - Servings: 16

Ingredients

- 16 oz. walnuts
- ½ c. butter

- ½ c. maple syrup, sugar-free
- 1 tbsp. vanilla extract, pure

Directions

1. Add all the ingredients into the Slow Cooker and turn it to low.
2. Cook for 2 hours stirring occasionally to ensure all the nuts are well coated.
3. When the time has elapsed, transfer the walnuts onto parchment paper. Let sit for a few minutes to cool.
4. Serve and enjoy.

Nutrition

- Calories: 328
- Total fat: 24 g.
- Saturated fat: 6 g.
- Total carbohydrates: 10 g.
- Net carbohydrates: 8 g.

- Protein: 4 g.
- Sugar: 7 g.
- Fiber: 2 g.
- Sodium: 2 mg.
- Potassium: 127 g.

3.8   HAM AND CHEESE STRATA

Preparation time: 10 minutes - Cooking time: 3 hours - Servings: 6

Ingredients

- 1 tbsp. butter
- 8 slices low-carb Ezekiel bread divided into 16 triangles remove crust and save
- 6 oz. thinly sliced ham, chopped
- 8 oz. Monterey jack cheese, shredded,
- 2 tbsp. minced onions, dried

- 6 eggs
- 3 ¼ c. half-and-half
- ½ tbsp. salt
- ¼ tbsp. tabasco sauce
- ¾ tbsp. black pepper

Directions

1. Grease your Slow Cooker with butter then put 8 triangles of bread at the bottom. Sprinkle the trimmed-off crust pieces to fully cover the bottom of your Slow Cooker with bread.
2. Sprinkle ham over the bread to make a thick layer, then add cheese preserving ½ c.
3. Sprinkle half of the onions over cheese then top with remaining bread slices. Set aside.
4. Mix eggs, half-and-half, salt, tabasco sauce, and pepper in a mixing bowl until well blended.
5. Pour the egg mixture over the bread then sprinkle the remaining onions on top. Let sit for about 15 minutes.
6. Sprinkle reserved cheese and cover your Slow Cooker.
7. Cook for about 3 hours on low and when time has elapsed, uncover your Slow Cooker.
8. Let the strata sit for about 10 minutes before cutting.
9. Serve and enjoy.

Nutrition

- Calories: 481.4
- Total fat: 37.8 g.
- Saturated fat: 20.5 g.
- Total carbohydrates: 11.4 g.
- Protein: 23.9 g.
- Sugar: 1.1 g.
- Fiber: 1 g.
- Potassium: 382 mg.
- Sodium: 1,334 mg.

3.9   TEXAS TOAST CASSEROLE

Preparation time: 10 minutes - Cooking time: 30 minutes - Servings: 10

Ingredients

- ½ c. butter, melted
- 1 c. brown Swerve
- 1 lb. Texas Toast bread, sliced
- 4 large eggs
- 1 ½ c. milk
- 1 tbsp. vanilla extract
- 2 tbsps. Swerve
- 2 tsps. cinnamon
- Maple syrup for serving

Directions

1. Layer a 9x13-inch baking pan with cooking spray.
2. Spread the bread slices at the bottom of the prepared pan.
3. Whisk the eggs with the remaining ingredients in a mixer.
4. Pour this mixture over the bread slices evenly.
5. Bake the bread for 30 minutes at 350°F in a preheated oven.
6. Serve.

Nutrition

- Calories: 332
- Total fat: 13.7 g.
- Sodium: 350 mg.
- Dietary fiber: 2 g.
- Sugar: 6 g.
- Protein: 7.4 g.

- Calcium: 143 mg.
- Phosphorus: 186 mg.
- Potassium: 74 mg.

3.10 SUPER SCRAMBLED EGGS

Preparation time: 10 minutes - Cooking time: 10 minutes - Servings: 2

Ingredients

- ½ c. cream cheese
- ¼ c. unsweetened almond or rice milk
- 3 eggs
- 2 egg whites
- 1 tbsp. finely chopped scallion, green part only
- 2 tbsps. unsalted butter
- 1 tbsp. chopped fresh tarragon
- Ground black pepper, to taste

Directions

1. In a mixing bowl, whisk eggs and whites. Add cream cheese, milk, scallions, and tarragon. Combine to mix well with each other.
2. Take a medium saucepan or skillet, add butter. Heat over medium heat.
3. Add egg mixture and stir-cook for 4–5 minutes until eggs are scrambled evenly.
4. Season with black pepper, and serve warm.

Nutrition

- Calories: 238
- Fat: 17 g.
- Phosphorus: 117 mg.
- Potassium: 152 mg.
- Sodium: 211 mg.
- Carbohydrates: 3 g.
- Protein: 8 g.

3.11 MUSHROOM TOFU BREAKFAST

Preparation time: 10 minutes - Cooking time: 10 minutes - Servings: 2

Ingredients

- 1 tbsp. chopped shallots
- ½ c. sliced white mushrooms
- ⅓ c. medium-firm tofu, crumbled
- ⅓ tsp. turmeric
- 1 tsp. cumin
- ⅓ tsp. smoked paprika
- 3 tbsps. vegetable oil 1 pinch of garlic salt
- Pepper

Directions

1. Take a medium saucepan or skillet, add oil. Heat over medium heat.
2. Add shallots, mushrooms, and stir-cook until they become softened for 3–4 minutes.
3. Add tofu, salt, spices, and stir-cook until tofu is tender and cooked well.
4. Serve warm.

Nutrition

- Calories: 217
- Fat: 21 g.
- Phosphorus: 77 mg.
- Potassium: 147 mg.
- Sodium: 301 mg.
- Carbohydrates: 3 g.
- Protein: 4 g.

3.12 HERBED OMELET

Preparation time: 5 minutes - Cooking time: 10 minutes - Servings: 2

Ingredients

- 4 eggs
- 2 tbsps. water
- 1 ½ tsps. vegetable oil
- 1 tbsp. chopped onion
- ¼ tsp. basil
- ⅛ tsp. tarragon
- ¼ tsp. parsley (optional)

Directions

1. Take a mixing bowl and beat eggs. Add water and spices; combine.
2. Take a medium saucepan or skillet, add oil. Heat over medium heat.
3. Add onion and stir-cook until become translucent and softened. Set aside.
4. Add the egg mixture into the pan and spread evenly.
5. Cook over both sides until well set and lightly brown.
6. Serve warm with cooked onions on top.

Nutrition

- Calories: 204
- Fat: 14 g.
- Phosphorus: 201 mg.
- Potassium: 166 mg.
- Sodium: 174 mg.
- Carbohydrates: 1 g.
- Protein: 14 g.

3.13 WHOLESOME PANCAKES

Preparation time: 10 minutes - Cooking time: 20 minutes - Servings: 2

Ingredients

- ¼ tsp. ground cinnamon
- 1 pinch of ground nutmeg
- 2 eggs
- ½ c. unsweetened almond or rice milk
- ½ c. all-purpose flour

Directions

1. Preheat an oven to 450°F.
2. In a mixing bowl, add milk and eggs. Whisk to mix well with each other.

3. Add flour, cinnamon, and nutmeg; combine to blend well.
4. Take an oven-proof skillet; grease with some cooking spray.
5. Spread's batter over it evenly and bake for about 20 minutes until you see crisp edges, and puffed up.
6. Slice in halves, and serve warm.

Nutrition

- Calories: 173
- Fat: 1 g.
- Phosphorus: 85 mg.
- Potassium: 122 mg.

- Sodium: 51 mg.
- Carbohydrates: 28 g.
- Protein: 7 g.

3.14 HEALTHY CEREAL BREAKFAST

Preparation time: 10 minutes - Cooking time: 20 minutes - Servings: 2

Ingredients

- 6 tbsps. uncooked bulgur
- 2 tbsps. uncooked whole buckwheat
- 2 ¼ c. water
- 1 ¼ c. vanilla rice milk

- 6 tbsps. plain uncooked couscous
- ½ tsp. ground cinnamon
- 1 c. peeled, sliced apple

Directions

1. Take a medium saucepan, heat milk and water over medium-high heat.
2. Add bulgur, buckwheat, and apple; stir the mixture.
3. Over low heat, simmer the mixture for about 20–25 minutes, stir in between, until cereal is tender.
4. Take off heat; mix in cinnamon and couscous.
5. Cover and set aside for 10 minutes.
6. Fluff mixture, and serve warm.

Nutrition

- Calories: 174
- Fat: 2 g.
- Phosphorus: 127 mg.
7. Protein: 4 g.

- Potassium: 134 mg.
- Sodium: 62 mg.
- Carbohydrates: 31 g.

3.15 BREAKFAST SALAD FROM GRAINS AND FRUITS

Preparation time: 5 minutes - Cooking time: 15 minutes - Servings: 2

Ingredients

- 1 8 oz. low-fat vanilla yogurt
- 1 c. raisins
- 1 orange
- 1 Red Delicious apple
- 1 Granny Smith apple
- ¾ c. bulgur
- ¾ c. quick-cooking brown rice
- ¼ tsp. salt
- 3 c. water

Directions

1. On high fire, place a large pot and bring water to a boil.
2. Add bulgur and rice. Lower fire to a simmer and cooks for 10 minutes while covered.
3. Turn off fire, set aside for 2 minutes while covered.
4. In a baking sheet, transfer, and evenly spread grains to cool.
5. Meanwhile, peel orange and cut it into units. Chop and core apples.
6. Once grains are cool, transfer to a large serving bowl along with fruits.
7. Add yogurt and mix well to coat.
8. Serve and enjoy.

Nutrition

- Calories: 187
- Carbohydrates: 6 g.
- Protein: 4 g.
- Fat: 4 g.
- Phosphorus: 69 mg.
- Potassium: 88 mg.
- Sodium: 117 mg.

3.16 FRENCH TOAST WITH APPLESAUCE

Preparation time: 5 minutes - Cooking time: 15 minutes - Servings: 2

Ingredients

- ¼ c. unsweetened applesauce
- ½ c. milk
- 1 tsp. ground cinnamon
- 2 eggs
- 2 tbsp. white sugar
- 6 slices whole wheat bread

Directions

1. Mix well applesauce, sugar, cinnamon, milk, and eggs in a mixing bowl.
2. Soak the bread, one by one into the applesauce mixture until wet.
3. On medium fire, heat a nonstick skillet greased with cooking spray.
4. Add soaked bread one at a time and cook for 2–3 minutes per side or until lightly browned.
5. Serve and enjoy.

Nutrition

- Calories: 57
- Carbohydrates: 6 g.
- Protein: 4 g.
- Fat: 4 g.

- Phosphorus: 69 mg.
- Potassium: 88 mg.
- Sodium: 43 mg.

3.17 BAGELS MADE HEALTHY

Preparation time: 5 minutes - Cooking time: 25 minutes - Servings: 2

Ingredients

- 2 tsp. yeast
- 1 ½ tbsp. olive oil
- 1 ¼ c. bread flour
- 2 c. whole wheat flour

- 1 tbsp. vinegar
- 2 tbsp. honey
- 1 ½ c. warm water

Directions

1. In a bread machine, mix all ingredients, and then process on dough cycle.
2. Once done or end of the cycle, create 8 pieces shaped like a flattened ball.
3. In the center of each ball, make a hole using your thumb then create a donut shape.
4. In a greased baking sheet, place donut-shaped dough then covers and let it rise about ½ hour.
5. Prepare about 2-inch of water to boil in a large pan.
6. In boiling water, drop one at a time the bagels and boil for 1 minute, then turn them once.
7. Remove them and return them to a baking sheet and bake at 350°F (175°C) for about 20–25 minutes until golden brown.

Nutrition

- Calories: 221
- Carbohydrates: 42 g.
- Protein: 7 g.
- Sodium: 47 mg.

- Fat: 3 g
- Phosphorus: 130 mg.
- Potassium: 166 mg.

3.18 CORNBREAD WITH SOUTHERN TWIST

Preparation time: 15 minutes - Cooking time: 60 minutes - Servings: 2

Ingredients

- 2 tbsps. shortening
- 1 ¼ c. skim milk
- ¼ c. egg substitute
- 4 tbsps. sodium-free baking powder
- ½ c. flour
- 1 ½ c. cornmeal

Directions

1. Prepare an 8x8-inch baking dish or a black iron skillet then add shortening.
2. Put the baking dish or skillet inside the oven at 425°F, once the shortening has melted that means the pan is hot already.
3. In a bowl, add milk and egg then mix well.
4. Add flour, baking powder, and cornmeal.
5. Take out the skillet and add the melted shortening into the batter and stir well.
6. Pour all mixed ingredients into a skillet.
7. For 15–20 minutes, cook in the oven until golden brown.

Nutrition

- Calories: 166
- Carbohydrates: 35 g.
- Protein: 5 g.
- Fat: 1 g.
- Phosphorus: 79 mg.
- Potassium: 122 mg.
- Sodium: 34 mg.

3.19 GRANDMA'S PANCAKE SPECIAL

Preparation time: 5 minutes - Cooking time: 15 minutes- Servings: 3

Ingredients

- 1 tbsp. oil
- 1 c. milk
- 1 egg
- 2 tsps. sodium-free baking powder
- 2 tbsps. sugar
- 1 ¼ c. flour

Directions

1. Mix together all the dry ingredients such as the flour, sugar, and baking powder.
2. Combine oil, milk, and egg in another bowl. Once done, add them all to the flour mixture.
3. Make sure that as your stir the mixture, blend them together until slightly lumpy.
4. In a hot greased griddle, pour in at least ¼ c. of the batter to make each pancake.
5. To cook, ensure that the bottom is a bit brown, then turn and cook the other side, as well.

Nutrition

- Calories: 167
- Carbohydrates: 50 g.
- Protein: 11 g.
- Fat: 11 g.

- Phosphorus: 176 mg.
- Potassium: 215 mg.
- Sodium: 70 mg.

3.20   GRILLED CHICKEN POWER BOWL WITH GREEN GODDESS DRESSING

Preparation time: 5 minutes - Cooking time: 15 minutes - Servings: 4

Ingredients

- 1 ½ boneless, skinless chicken breasts
- ¼ tsp. each salt and pepper
- 1 c. rice or cubed kabocha squash
- 1 c. diced zucchini
- 1 c. rice yellow summer squash

- 1 c. rice broccoli
- 8 cherry tomatoes, halved
- 4 radishes, sliced thin
- 1 c. shredded red cabbage
- ¼ c. hemp or pumpkin seeds

For the green goddess dressing:

- ½ c. low-fat plain Greek yogurt
- 1 c. fresh basil
- 1 clove garlic

- 4 tbsp. lemon juice
- ¼ tsp. salt
- ¼ tsp. pepper

Directions

1. Preheat oven to 350°F.
2. Season chicken with salt and pepper.
3. Roast chicken for 12 minutes until it reaches a temperature of 165°F. When done, dismiss from the oven and set aside to rest for about 5 minutes. Cut into bite-sized pieces and keep warm.
4. While the chicken rests, steam riced kabocha squash, yellow summer squash, zucchini, and broccoli in a covered microwave-proof bowl for about 5 minutes till tender.
5. For the dressing, arrange the ingredients in a blender and puree till smooth.
6. To serve, place an equal amount of veggie mix into 4 individual bowls. Add an equal amount of cherry tomatoes, radishes, and chopped cabbage to each bowl along with ¼ of the chicken and 1 tbsp. of seeds. Dress up. Enjoy!

Nutrition

- Calories: 300
- Protein: 43 g.
- Fat: 10 g.

- Carbohydrates: 12 g.

CHAPTER 4 - LUNCH RECIPES

4.1   SALAD WITH VINAIGRETTE

Preparation time: 25 minutes - Cooking time: 0 minutes - Servings: 4

Ingredients

For the vinaigrette:

- ½ c. olive oil
- 4 tbsps. balsamic vinegar
- 2 tbsps. chopped fresh oregano
- 1 pinch of red pepper flakes
- Ground black pepper

For the salad:

- 4 c. shredded green leaf lettuce
- 1 carrot, shredded
- ¾ c. fresh green beans, cut into 1-inch pieces
- 3 large radishes, sliced thin

Directions

1. To make the vinaigrette: Put the vinaigrette ingredients in a bowl and whisk.
2. To make the salad: In a bowl, toss together the carrot, lettuce, green beans, and radishes.
3. Add the vinaigrette to the vegetables and toss to coat.
4. Arrange the salad on plates and serve.

Nutrition

- Calories: 273
- Fat: 27 g.
- Carbohydrates: 7 g.
- Phosphorus: 30 mg.
- Potassium: 197 mg.
- Sodium: 27 mg.
- Protein: 1 g.

4.2 SALAD WITH LEMON DRESSING

Preparation time: 10 minutes -Cooking time: 0 minutes - Servings: 4

Ingredients

- ¼ c. heavy cream
- ¼ c. freshly squeezed lemon juice
- 2 tbsps. granulated sugar
- 2 tbsps. chopped fresh dill
- 2 tbsps. finely chopped scallion, green part only
- ¼ tsp. ground black pepper
- 1 English cucumber, sliced thin
- 2 c. shredded green cabbage

Directions

1. In a small bowl, stir together the lemon juice, cream, sugar, dill, scallion, and pepper until well blended.
2. In a large bowl, toss together the cucumber and cabbage.
3. Place the salad in the refrigerator and chill for 1 hour.
4. Stir before serving.

Nutrition

- Calories: 99
- Fat: 6 g.
- Carbohydrates: 13 g.
- Phosphorus: 38 mg.
- Potassium: 200 mg.
- Sodium: 14 mg.
- Protein: 2 g.

4.3 SHRIMP WITH SALSA

Preparation time: 15 minutes - Cooking time: 10 minutes - Servings: 4

Ingredients

- 2 tbsp. olive oil
- 6 oz. large shrimp, peeled and deveined, tails left on
- 1 tsp. minced garlic
- ½ c. chopped English cucumber
- ½ c. chopped mango
- Zest of 1 lime
- Juice of 1 lime
- Ground black pepper
- Lime wedges for garnish

Directions

1. Soak 4 wooden skewers in water for 30 minutes.
2. Preheat the barbecue to medium heat.
3. In a bowl, toss together the olive oil, shrimp, and garlic.
4. Thread the shrimp onto the skewers, about 4 shrimp per skewer.
5. In a bowl, stir together the mango, cucumber, lime zest, and lime juice, and season the salsa lightly with pepper. Set aside.
6. Grill the shrimp for 10 minutes, turning once or until the shrimp is opaque and cooked through.
7. Season the shrimp lightly with pepper.

8. Serve the shrimp on the cucumber salsa with lime wedges on the side.

Nutrition

- Calories: 120
- Fat: 8 g.
- Carbohydrates: 4 g.
- Phosphorus: 91 mg.

- Potassium: 129 mg.
- Sodium: 60 mg.
- Protein: 9 g.

4.4 CAULIFLOWER SOUP

Preparation time: 30 minutes - Cooking time: 30 minutes - Servings: 6

Ingredients

- 1 tsp. unsalted butter
- 1 small sweet onion, chopped
- 2 tsps. minced garlic
- 1 small head cauliflower, cut into small florets

- 2 tsps. curry powder
- Water to cover the cauliflower
- ½ c. light sour cream
- 3 tbsps. chopped fresh cilantro

Directions

1. In a large saucepan, heat the butter over medium-high heat and sauté onion and garlic for about 3 minutes or until softened.
2. Add the cauliflower, water, and curry powder.
3. Bring the soup to a boil, then reduce the heat to low and simmer for 20 minutes or until the cauliflower is tender.
4. Puree the soup until creamy and smooth with a hand mixer.
5. Transfer the soup back into a saucepan and stir in the sour cream and cilantro.
6. Heat the soup on medium heat for 5 minutes or until warmed through.

Nutrition

- Calories: 33
- Fat: 2 g.
- Carbohydrates: 4 g.
- Protein: 1 g.

- Phosphorus: 30 mg.
- Potassium: 167 mg.
- Sodium: 22 mg.

4.5 CABBAGE STEW

Preparation time: 20 minutes - Cooking time: 34 minutes - Servings: 6

Ingredients

- 1 tsp. unsalted butter
- ½ large sweet onion, chopped
- 1 tsp. minced garlic
- 6 c. shredded green cabbage
- 3 celery stalks, chopped with leafy tops
- 1 scallion, both green and white parts, chopped
- 2 tbsps. chopped fresh parsley

- 2 tbsps. freshly squeezed lemon juice
- 1 tbsp. chopped fresh thyme
- 1 tsp. chopped savory
- 1 tsp. chopped fresh oregano
- Water
- 1 c. fresh green beans, cut into 1-inch pieces
- Ground black pepper

Directions

1. Melt the butter in a pot.
2. Sauté the onion and garlic in the melted butter for 3 minutes, or until the vegetables are softened.
3. Add the celery, cabbage, scallion, parsley, lemon juice, thyme, savory, and oregano to the pot, add enough water to cover the vegetables by 4-inch.
4. Bring the soup to a boil. Reduce the heat to low and simmer the soup for 25 minutes or until the vegetables are tender.
5. Add the green beans and simmer for 3 minutes.
6. Season with pepper.

Nutrition

- Calories: 33
- Fat: 1 g.
- Carbohydrates: 6 g.
- Phosphorus: 29 mg.

- Potassium: 187 mg.
- Sodium: 20 mg.
- Protein: 1 g.

4.6 BAKED HADDOCK

Preparation time: 10 minutes - Cooking time: 20 minutes - Servings: 4

Ingredients

- ½ c. breadcrumbs
- 3 tbsps. chopped fresh parsley
- 1 tbsp. lemon zest
- 1 tsp. chopped fresh thyme

- ¼ tsp. ground black pepper
- 1 tbsp. melted unsalted butter
- 12 oz. haddock fillets, deboned and skinned

Directions

1. Preheat the oven to 350F.
2. In a bowl, stir together the parsley, breadcrumbs, lemon zest, thyme, and pepper until well combined.

3. Add the melted butter and toss until the mixture resembles coarse crumbs.
4. Place the haddock on a baking sheet and spoon the breadcrumb mixture on top, pressing down firmly.
5. Bake the haddock in the oven for 20 minutes or until the fish is just cooked through and flakes off in chunks when pressed.

Nutrition

- Calories: 143
- Fat: 4 g.
- Carbohydrates: 10 g.
- Phosphorus: 216 mg.

- Potassium: 285 mg.
- Sodium: 281 mg.
- Protein: 16 g.

4.7 HERBED CHICKEN

Preparation time: 20 minutes - Cooking time: 15 minutes - Servings: 4

Ingredients

- 12 oz. chicken breast boneless, skinless, and cut into 8 strips
- 1 egg white
- 2 tbsps. water, divided
- ½ c. breadcrumbs
- ¼ c. unsalted butter, divided

- Juice of 1 lemon
- Zest of 1 lemon
- 1 tbsp. fresh chopped basil
- 1 tsp. fresh chopped thyme
- Lemon slices, for garnish

Directions

1. Place the chicken strips between 2 sheets of plastic wrap and pound each flat with a rolling pin.
2. In a bowl, whisk together the egg and 1 tbsp. of water.
3. Put the breadcrumbs in another bowl.
4. Dredge the chicken strips, one at a time, in the egg, then into the breadcrumbs, and set the breaded strips aside on a plate.
5. In a large skillet over medium heat, melt 2 tbsps. of the butter.
6. Cook the strips in the butter for 3 minutes, turning once, or until they are golden and cooked through. Transfer the chicken to a plate.
7. Add the lemon zest, lemon juice, basil, thyme, and the remaining 1 tbsp. of water to the skillet and stir until the mixture simmers.
8. Remove the sauce from the heat and stir in the remaining 2 tbsps. butter.
9. Serve the chicken with the lemon sauce drizzled over the top and garnished with lemon slices.

Nutrition

- Calories: 255
- Fat: 14 g.
- Carbohydrates: 11 g.
- Phosphorus: 180 mg.

- Potassium: 321 mg.
- Sodium: 261 mg.
- Protein: 20 g.

4.8 PESTO PORK CHOPS

Preparation time: 20 minutes - Cooking time: 20 minutes - Servings: 4

Ingredients

- 4 (3 oz.) pork top-loin chops boneless, fat-trimmed
- 8 tsps. herb pesto
- ½ c. breadcrumbs
- 1 tbsp. olive oil

Directions

1. Preheat the oven to 450F.
2. Line a baking sheet with foil. Set aside.
3. Rub 1 tsp. of pesto evenly over both sides of each pork chop.
4. Lightly dredge each pork chop in the breadcrumbs.
5. Heat the oil in a skillet.
6. Brown the pork chops on each side for 5 minutes.
7. Place the pork chops on the baking sheet.
8. Bake for 10 minutes or until pork reaches 145°F in the center.

Nutrition

- Calories: 210
- Fat: 7 g.
- Carbohydrates: 10 g.
- Phosphorus: 179 mg.
- Potassium: 220 mg.
- Sodium: 148 mg.
- Protein: 24 g.

4.9 VEGETABLE CURRY

Preparation time: 15 minutes - Cooking time: 45 minutes - Servings: 4

Ingredients

- 2 tsps. olive oil
- ½ sweet onion, diced
- 2 tsps. minced garlic
- 2 tsps. grated fresh ginger
- ½ eggplant, peeled and diced
- 1 carrot, peeled and diced
- 1 red bell pepper, diced
- 1 tbsp. hot curry powder
- 1 tsp. ground cumin
- ½ tsp. coriander
- 1 pinch of cayenne pepper
- 1 ½ c. homemade vegetable stock
- 1 tbsp. cornstarch
- ¼ c. water

Directions

1. Heat the oil in a stockpot.
2. Sauté the ginger, garlic, and onion for 3 minutes or until they are softened.
3. Add the red pepper, carrots, eggplant, and stir often for 6 minutes.
4. Stir in the cumin, curry powder, coriander, cayenne pepper, and vegetable stock.

5. Bring the curry to a boil and then lower the heat to low.

6. Simmer the curry for 30 minutes or until the vegetables are tender.

7. In a bowl, stir together the cornstarch and water.

8. Stir in the cornstarch mixture into the curry and simmer for 5 minutes or until the sauce has thickened.

Nutrition

- Calories: 100
- Fat: 3 g.
- Carbohydrates: 9 g.
- Phosphorus: 28 mg.

- Potassium: 180 mg.
- Sodium: 218 mg.
- Protein: 1 g.

4.10 GRILLED STEAK WITH SALSA

Preparation time: 20 minutes - Cooking time: 15 minutes - Servings: 4

Ingredients

For the salsa:

- 1 c. English cucumber, chopped
- ¼ c. red bell pepper, boiled and diced
- 1 scallion, both green and white parts, chopped

- 2 tbsps. fresh cilantro, chopped
- Juice of 1 lime

For the steak:

- 4 (3 oz.) beef tenderloin steaks, room temperature

- Olive oil
- Freshly ground black pepper

Directions

1. To make the salsa: In a bowl, combine the lime juice, cilantro, scallion, bell pepper, and cucumber. Set aside.

2. To make the steak: Preheat a barbecue to medium heat.

3. Rub the steaks all over with oil and season with pepper.

4. Grill the steaks for about 5 minutes per side for medium-rare, or until the desired doneness.

5. Serve the steaks topped with salsa.

Nutrition

- Calories: 130
- Fat: 6 g.
- Carbohydrates: 1 g.
- Protein: 19 g.

- Phosphorus: 186 mg.
- Potassium: 272 mg.
- Sodium: 39 mg.

4.11   BUFFALO CHICKEN LETTUCE WRAPS

Preparation time: 35 minutes - Cooking time: 10 minutes - Servings: 2

Ingredients

- 3 chicken breasts, boneless and cubed
- 20 slices of almond butter lettuce leaves
- ¾ c. cherry tomatoes halved
- ¼ c. green onions, diced
- ½ c. ranch dressing
- ¾ c. hot sauce

Directions

1. Take a mixing bowl and add chicken cubes and hot sauce, mix.
2. Place in the fridge and let it marinate for 30 minutes.
3. Preheat your oven to 400°F.
4. Place coated chicken on a cookie pan and bake for 9 minutes.
5. Assemble lettuce serving cups with equal amounts of lettuce, green onions, tomatoes, ranch dressing, and cubed chicken.
6. Serve and enjoy!

Nutrition

- Calories: 106
- Fat: 6 g.
- Net carbohydrates: 2 g.
- Protein: 5 g.
- Phosphorus: 216 mg.
- Potassium: 285 mg.
- Sodium: 281 mg.
- Protein: 16 g.

4.12   CRAZY JAPANESE POTATO AND BEEF CROQUETTES

Preparation time: 10 minutes - Cooking time: 20 minutes - Servings: 10

Ingredients

- 3 medium russet potatoes, peeled and chopped
- 1 tbsp. almond butter
- 1 tbsp. vegetable oil
- 3 onions, diced
- ¾ lb. ground beef
- 4 tsps. light coconut aminos
- All-purpose flour for coating
- 2 eggs, beaten
- Panko breadcrumbs for coating
- ½ c. oil, frying
- ½ cup Sunflower seeds water

Directions

1. Take a saucepan and place it over medium-high heat; add potatoes and sunflower seeds water, boil for 16 minutes.
2. Remove water and put potatoes in another bowl, add almond butter and mash the potatoes.
3. Take a frying pan and place it over medium heat, add 1 tbsp. oil and let it heat up.
4. Add onions and stir fry until tender.
5. Add coconut aminos to beef.
6. Keep frying until beef is browned.

7. Mix the beef with the potatoes evenly.
8. Take another frying pan and place it over medium heat; add ½ c. of oil.
9. Form croquettes using the mashed potato mixture and coat them with flour, then eggs, and finally breadcrumbs.
10. Fry patties until golden on all sides.

Nutrition

- Calories: 239
- Fat: 4 g.
- Carbohydrates: 20 g.
- Protein: 10 g.

- Phosphorus: 116 mg.
- Potassium: 225 mg.
- Sodium: 181 mg.

4.13 SAUCY GARLIC GREENS

Preparation time: 5 minutes - Cooking time: 20 minutes - Servings: 4

Ingredients

- 1 bunch of leafy greens

For the sauce:

- ½ c. cashews soaked in water for 10 minutes
- ¼ c. water
- 1 tbsp. lemon juice

- 1 tsp. coconut aminos
- 1 clove garlic, peeled
- ⅛ tsp. flavored vinegar

Directions

1. Make the sauce by draining and discarding the soaking water from your cashews and add the cashews to a blender.
2. Add fresh water, lemon juice, flavored vinegar, coconut aminos, garlic.
3. Blitz until you have a smooth cream and transfer to a bowl.
4. Add ½ c. of water to the pot.
5. Place the steamer basket to the pot and add the greens into the basket.
6. Lock the lid and steam for 1 minute.
7. Quick-release the pressure.
8. Transfer the steamed greens to a strainer and extract excess water.
9. Place the greens into a mixing bowl.
10. Add lemon-garlic sauce and toss.

Nutrition

- Calories: 77
- Fat: 5 g.
- Carbohydrates: 0 g.
- Protein: 2 g.
- Phosphorus: 126 mg.

- Potassium: 255 mg.
- Sodium: 281 mg.

4.14 GARDEN SALAD

Preparation time: 5 minutes - Cooking time: 20 minutes - Servings: 6

Ingredients

- 1 lb. raw peanuts in the shell
- 1 bay leaf
- 2 medium-sized chopped-up tomatoes
- ½ c. diced up green pepper
- ½ c. diced up sweet onion
- ¼ c. finely diced hot pepper
- ¼ c. diced up celery
- 2 tbsps. olive oil
- ¾ tsp. flavored vinegar
- ¼ tsp. freshly ground black pepper

Directions

1. Boil your peanuts for 1 minute and rinse them.
2. The skin will be soft, so discard the skin.
3. Add 2 c. of water to the Instant Pot.
4. Add bay leaf and peanuts.
5. Lock the lid and cook on high pressure for 20 minutes.
6. Drain the water.
7. Take a large bowl and add the peanuts and diced vegetables.
8. Whisk in olive oil, flavored vinegar, pepper in another bowl.
9. Pour the mixture over the salad and mix.

Nutrition

- Calories: 140
- Fat: 4 g.
- Carbohydrates: 24 g.
- Protein: 5 g.
- Phosphorus: 216 mg.
- Potassium: 185 mg.
- Sodium: 141 mg.

4.15 SPICY CABBAGE DISH

Preparation time: 10 minutes - Cooking time: 4 hours - Servings: 4

Ingredients

- 2 yellow onions, chopped
- 10 c. red cabbage, shredded
- 1 c. plums, pitted and chopped
- 1 tsp. cinnamon powder
- 1 garlic clove, minced
- 1 tsp. cumin seeds
- ¼ tsp. cloves, ground
- 2 tbsps. red wine vinegar
- 1 tsp. coriander seeds
- ½ c. water

Directions

1. Add cabbage, onion, plums, garlic, cumin, cinnamon, cloves, vinegar, coriander, and water to your Slow Cooker.
2. Stir well.
3. Place lid and cook on low for 4 hours.

4. Divide between serving platters.

Nutrition

- Calories: 197
- Fat: 1 g.
- Carbohydrates: 14 g.
- Protein: 3 g.

- Phosphorus: 216 mg.
- Potassium: 285 mg.
- Sodium: 281 mg.

4.16 EXTREME BALSAMIC CHICKEN

Preparation time: 10 minutes - Cooking time: 35 minutes - Servings: 4

Ingredients

- 3 boneless chicken breasts, skinless
- Sunflower seeds to taste
- ¼ c. almond flour
- ⅔ c. low-fat chicken broth

- 1 ½ tsps. arrowroot
- ½ c. low-sugar raspberry preserve
- 1 ½ tbsps. balsamic vinegar

Directions

1. Cut chicken breast into bite-sized pieces and season them with seeds.
2. Dredge the chicken pieces in flour and shake off any excess.
3. Take a nonstick skillet and place it over medium heat.
4. Add chicken to the skillet and cook for 15 minutes, making sure to turn them halfway through.
5. Remove chicken and transfer to a platter.
6. Add arrowroot, broth, raspberry preserve to the skillet and stir.
7. Stir in balsamic vinegar and reduce heat to low, stir-cook for a few minutes.
8. Transfer the chicken back to the sauce and cook for 15 minutes more.
9. Serve and enjoy!

Nutrition

- Calories: 546
- Fat: 35 g.
- Carbohydrates: 11 g.
- Sodium: 81 mg.

- Protein: 44 g.
- Phosphorus: 136 mg.
- Potassium: 195 mg.

4.17 ENJOYABLE SPINACH AND BEAN MEDLEY

Preparation time: 10 minutes - Cooking time: 4 hours - Servings: 4

Ingredients

- 5 carrots, sliced
- 1 ½ c. great northern beans, dried
- 2 garlic cloves, minced
- 1 yellow onion, chopped
- Pepper to taste
- ½ tsp. oregano, dried
- 5 oz. baby spinach
- 4 ½ c. low-sodium veggie stock
- 2 tsps. lemon peel, grated
- 3 tbsp. lemon juice

Directions

1. Add beans, onion, carrots, garlic, oregano, pepper, and stock to your Slow Cooker.
2. Stir well.
3. Place lid and cook on high for 4 hours.
4. Add spinach, lemon juice, and lemon peel.
5. Stir and let it sit for 5 minutes.
6. Divide between serving platters and enjoy!

Nutrition

- Calories: 219
- Fat: 8 g.
- Carbohydrates: 14 g.
- Protein: 8 g.
- Phosphorus: 216 mg.
- Potassium: 285 mg.
- Sodium: 131 mg.

4.18 TANTALIZING CAULIFLOWER AND DILL MASH

Preparation time: 10 minutes - Cooking time: 6 hours - Servings: 6

Ingredients

- 1 cauliflower head, florets separated
- ⅓ c. dill, chopped
- 6 garlic cloves
- 2 tbsps. olive oil
- 1 pinch of black pepper

Directions

1. Add cauliflower to Slow Cooker.
2. Add dill, garlic, and water to cover them.
3. Place lid and cook on high for 5 hours.
4. Drain the flowers.
5. Season with pepper and add oil and mash using a potato masher.
6. Whisk and serve.

Nutrition

- Calories: 207
- Fat: 4 g.

- Carbohydrates: 14 g.
- Protein: 3 g.
- Phosphorus: 226 mg.
- Potassium: 285 mg.
- Sodium: 134 mg.

4.19 SECRET ASIAN GREEN BEANS

Preparation time: 10 minutes - Cooking time: 2 hours - Servings: 10

Ingredients

- 16 c. green beans, halved
- 3 tbsps. olive oil
- ¼ c. tomato sauce, salt-free
- ½ c. coconut sugar
- ¾ tsp. low-sodium soy sauce
- 1 pinch of pepper

Directions

1. Add green beans, coconut sugar, pepper, tomato sauce, soy sauce, and oil to your Slow Cooker.
2. Stir well.
3. Place lid and cook on low for 3 hours.
4. Divide between serving platters and serve.
5. Enjoy!

Nutrition

- Calories: 200
- Fat: 4 g.
- Carbohydrates: 12 g.
- Sodium: 131 mg.
- Protein: 3 g.
- Phosphorus: 216 mg.
- Potassium: 285 mg.

4.20   EXCELLENT ACORN MIX

Preparation time: 10 minutes - Cooking time: 7 hours - Servings: 10

Ingredients

- 2 acorn squash, peeled and cut into wedges
- 16 oz. cranberry sauce, unsweetened
- ¼ tsp. cinnamon powder
- Pepper to taste
- Some Raisins

Directions

1. Add acorn wedges to your Slow Cooker.
2. Add cranberry sauce, cinnamon, raisins, and pepper.
3. Stir.
4. Place lid and cook on low for 7 hours.
5. Serve and enjoy!

Nutrition

- Calories: 200
- Fat: 3 g.
- Carbohydrates: 15 g.
- Protein: 2 g.
- Phosphorus: 211 mg.
- Potassium: 243 mg.
- Sodium: 203 mg.

CHAPTER 5 - DINNER RECIPES

5.1   MUSHROOM AND OLIVE MEDITERRANEAN STEAK

Preparation time: 10 minutes - Cooking time: 14 minutes - Servings: 2

Ingredients

- ½ lb. boneless beef sirloin steak, ¾-inch thick, cut into 4 pieces
- ½ large red onion, chopped
- ½ c. mushrooms
- 2 garlic cloves, thinly sliced
- 2 tbsps. olive oil
- ¼ c. green olives, coarsely chopped
- ½ c. parsley leaves, finely cut

Directions

1. Take a large-sized skillet and place it over medium-high heat.
2. Add oil and let it heat up.
3. Add beef and cook until both sides are browned, remove beef, and drain fat.
4. Add the rest of the oil to the skillet and heat.
5. Add onions, garlic and cook for 2–3 minutes.
6. Stir well.
7. Add mushrooms, olives and cook until the mushrooms are thoroughly done.
8. Return the beef to the skillet and reduce heat to medium.
9. Cook for 3–4 minutes (covered).
10. Stir in parsley.
11. Serve and enjoy!

Nutrition

- Calories: 386
- Fat: 30 g.
- Carbohydrates: 11 g.
- Protein: 21 g.

- Phosphorus: 296 mg.
- Potassium: 295 mg.
- Sodium: 111 mg.

5.2   HEARTY CHICKEN FRIED RICE

Preparation time: 10 minutes - Cooking time: 12 minutes - Servings: 4

Ingredients

- 1 tsp. olive oil
- 4 large egg whites
- 1 onion, chopped
- 2 garlic cloves, minced
- 12 oz. skinless chicken breasts, boneless, cut into ½-inch cubes

- ½ c. carrots, chopped
- ½ c. frozen green peas
- 2 c. long-grain brown rice, cooked
- 3 tbsps. soy sauce, low-sodium

Directions

1. Coat skillet with oil, place it over medium-high heat.
2. Add egg whites and cook until scrambled.
3. Sauté onion, garlic, and chicken breasts for 6 minutes.
4. Add carrots, peas and keep cooking for 3 minutes.
5. Stir in rice, season with soy sauce.
6. Add cooked egg whites, stir for 3 minutes.
7. Enjoy!

Nutrition

- Calories: 353
- Fat: 11 g.
- Carbohydrates: 30 g.
- Protein: 23 g.

- Phosphorus: 276 mg.
- Potassium: 295 mg.
- Sodium: 134 mg.

5.3   DECENT BEEF AND ONION STEW

Preparation time: 10 minutes - Cooking time: 1–2 hours - Servings: 4

Ingredients

- 2 lbs. lean beef, cubed
- 3 lbs. shallots, peeled
- 5 garlic cloves, peeled, whole
- 3 tbsps. tomato paste
- 1 bay leaves

- ¼ c. olive oil
- 3 tbsps. lemon juice

Directions

1. Take a stew pot and place it over medium heat.
2. Add olive oil and let it heat up.
3. Add meat and brown.
4. Add remaining ingredients and cover with water.
5. Bring the whole mix to a boil.
6. Reduce heat to low and cover the pot.
7. Simmer for 1–2 hours until beef is cooked thoroughly.
8. Serve hot!

Nutrition

- Calories: 136
- Fat: 3 g.
- Carbohydrates: 0.9 g.
- Protein: 24 g.

- Phosphorus: 396 mg.
- Potassium: 205 mg.
- Sodium: 141 mg.

5.4   CLEAN PARSLEY AND CHICKEN BREAST

Preparation time: 10 minutes - Cooking time: 40 minutes - Servings: 2

Ingredients

- ½ tbsp. dry parsley
- ½ tbsp. dry basil
- 2 chicken breast halves, boneless and skinless

- ¼ tsp. sunflower seeds
- ¼ tsp. red pepper flakes, crushed
- 1 tomato, sliced
- 1 Garlic, sliced

Directions

1. Preheat your oven to 350°F.
2. Take a 9x13-inch baking dish and grease it up with cooking spray.
3. Sprinkle 1 tbsp. of parsley, 1 tsp. of basil, and spread the mixture over your baking dish.
4. Arrange the chicken breast halves over the dish and sprinkle garlic slices on top.
5. Take a small bowl and add 1 tsp. parsley, 1 tsp. of basil, sunflower seeds, red pepper and mix well. Pour the mixture over the chicken breast.
6. Top with tomato slices and cover, bake for 25 minutes.
7. Remove the cover and bake for 15 minutes more.
8. Serve and enjoy!

Nutrition

- Calories: 150
- Fat: 4 g.
- Carbohydrates: 4 g.

- Protein: 25 g.
- Phosphorus: 196 mg.
- Potassium: 285 mg.

5.5 SODIUM: 111 MG. ZUCCHINI BEEF SAUTÉ WITH CORIANDER GREENS

Preparation time: 10 minutes - Cooking time: 10 minutes - Servings: 4

Ingredients

- 10 oz. beef, sliced into 1–2-inch strips
- 1 zucchini, cut into 2-inch strips
- ¼ c. parsley, chopped
- 3 garlic cloves, minced
- 2 tbsps. tamari sauce
- 4 tbsps. avocado oil

Directions

1. Add 2 tbsps. of avocado oil in a frying pan over high heat.
2. Place strips of beef and brown for a few minutes on high heat.
3. Once the meat is brown, add zucchini strips and sauté until tender.
4. Once tender, add tamari sauce, garlic, parsley and let them sit for a few minutes more.
5. Serve immediately and enjoy!

Nutrition

- Calories: 500
- Fat: 40 g.
- Carbohydrates: 5 g.
- Protein: 31 g.
- Phosphorus: 236 mg.
- Potassium: 249 mg.
- Sodium: 143 mg.

5.6 HEALTHY LEMON AND PEPPER CHICKEN

Preparation time: 5 minutes - Cooking time: 15 - Servings: 4

Ingredients

- 2 tsps. olive oil
- 1 ¼ lbs. skinless chicken cutlets
- 2 whole eggs
- ¼ c. panko crumbs
- 1 tbsp. lemon pepper
- Sunflower seeds
- Pepper to taste
- 3 c. green beans
- ¼ c. Parmesan cheese
- ¼ tsp. garlic powder

Directions

1. Preheat your oven to 425°F.
2. Take a bowl and stir in seasoning, Parmesan, lemon pepper, garlic powder, panko.
3. Whisk eggs in another bowl.
4. Coat cutlets in eggs and press into panko mix.
5. Transfer coated chicken to a parchment-lined baking sheet.
6. Toss the beans in oil, pepper, add sunflower seeds, and lay them on the side of the baking sheet.
7. Bake for 15 minutes.
8. Enjoy!

Nutrition

- Calories: 299
- Fat: 10 g.
- Carbohydrates: 10 g.
- Protein: 43 g.

- Phosphorus: 196 mg.
- Potassium: 285 mg.
- Sodium: 111 mg.

5.7   WALNUTS AND ASPARAGUS DELIGHT

Preparation time: 5 minutes - Cooking time: 5 minutes - Servings: 4

Ingredients

- 1 ½ tbsps. olive oil
- ¾ lb. asparagus, trimmed
- ¼ c. walnuts, chopped

- Sunflower seeds
- Pepper to taste

Directions

1. Place a skillet over medium heat add olive oil and let it heat up.
2. Add asparagus, sauté for 5 minutes until browned.
3. Season with sunflower seeds and pepper.
4. Remove heat.
5. Add walnuts and toss.
6. Serve warm!

Nutrition

- Calories: 124
- Fat: 12 g.
- Carbohydrates: 2 g.
- Sodium: 121 mg.

- Protein: 3 g.
- Phosphorus: 196 mg.
- Potassium: 205 mg.

5.8   HEALTHY CARROT CHIPS

Preparation time: 10 minutes - Cooking time: 10 minutes - Servings: 4

Ingredients

- 3 c. carrots, sliced paper-thin rounds
- 2 tbsps. olive oil
- 2 tsps. ground cumin
- ½ tsp. smoked paprika
- 1 pinch of sunflower seeds

Directions

1. Preheat your oven to 400°F.
2. Slice carrots into paper-thin-shaped coins using a peeler.
3. Place slices in a bowl and toss with oil and spices.
4. Lay out the slices on a parchment paper, lined baking sheet in a single layer.
5. Sprinkle sunflower seeds.
6. Transfer to oven and bake for 8–10 minutes.
7. Remove and serve.
8. Enjoy!

Nutrition

- Calories: 434
- Fat: 35 g.
- Carbohydrates: 31 g.
- Protein: 2 g.
- Phosphorus: 196 mg.
- Potassium: 285 mg.
- Sodium: 111 mg.

5.9   BEEF SOUP

Preparation time: 10 minutes - Cooking time: 40 minutes - Servings: 4

Ingredients

- 1 lb. ground beef, lean
- 1 c. mixed vegetables, frozen
- 1 yellow onion, chopped
- 6 c. vegetable broth
- 1 c. low-fat cream
- Pepper to taste
- ½ teaspoon Salt to taste

Directions

1. Take a Stockpot and add all the ingredients except heavy cream, salt, and black pepper.
2. Bring to a boil.
3. Reduce heat to simmer.
4. Cook for 40 minutes.
5. Once cooked, warm the heavy cream.
6. Then add once the soup is cooked.
7. Blend the soup till smooth by using an immersion blender.

8. Season with salt and black pepper.
9. Serve and enjoy!

Nutrition

- Calories: 270
- Fat: 14 g.
- Carbohydrates: 6 g.
- Protein: 29 g.

- Phosphorus: 187 mg.
- Potassium: 258 mg.
- Sodium: 145 mg.

5.10 AMAZING GRILLED CHICKEN AND BLUEBERRY SALAD

Preparation time: 10 minutes - Cooking time: 25 minutes - Servings: 5

Ingredients

- 5 c. mixed greens
- 1 c. blueberries

- ¼ c. slivered almonds
- 2 c. chicken breasts, cooked and cubed

For the dressing:

- ¼ c. olive oil
- ¼ c. apple cider vinegar
- ¼ c. blueberries

- 2 tbsps. honey
- Sunflower seeds and pepper to taste

Directions

1. Take a bowl and add greens, berries, almonds, chicken cubes and mix well.
2. Take a bowl and mix the dressing ingredients, pour the mix into a blender, and blitz until smooth.
3. Add dressing on top of the chicken cubes and toss well.
4. Season more and enjoy!

Nutrition

- Calories: 266
- Fat: 17 g.
- Carbohydrates: 18 g.
- Sodium: 91 mg.

- Protein: 10 g.
- Phosphorus: 196 mg.
- Potassium: 285 mg.

5.11 CLEAN CHICKEN AND MUSHROOM STEW

Preparation time: 10 minutes - Cooking time: 35 minutes - Servings: 4

Ingredients

- 4 chicken breast halves, cut into bite-sized pieces
- 1 lb. mushrooms, sliced (5–6 c.)
- 1 bunch spring onion, chopped
- 4 tbsps. olive oil
- 1 tsp. thyme
- Sunflower seeds and pepper as needed

Directions

1. Take a large deep-frying pan and place it over medium-high heat.
2. Add oil and let it heat up.
3. Add chicken and cook for 4–5 minutes per side until slightly browned.
4. Add spring onions and mushrooms, season with sunflower seeds, thyme, and pepper according to your taste.
5. Stir.
6. Cover with lid and bring the mix to a boil.
7. Reduce heat and simmer for 25 minutes.
8. Serve!

Nutrition

- Calories: 247
- Fat: 12 g.
- Carbohydrates: 10 g.
- Protein: 23 g.
- Phosphorus: 296 mg.
- Potassium: 215 mg.
- Sodium: 87 mg.

5.12 ELEGANT PUMPKIN CHILI DISH

Preparation time: 10 minutes - Cooking time: 15 minutes - Servings: 4

Ingredients

- 3 c. yellow onion, chopped
- 8 garlic cloves, chopped
- 1 lb. turkey, ground
- 2 cans (15 oz. each) fire-roasted tomatoes
- 2 c. pumpkin puree
- 1 c. chicken broth
- 4 tsps. chili spice
- 1 tsp. ground cinnamon
- 1 tsp. sea sunflower seeds
- 8 tsp. Coconut oil

Directions

1. Take a large-sized pot and place it over medium-high heat.
2. Add coconut oil and let the oil heat up.
3. Add onion and garlic, sauté for 5 minutes.
4. Add ground turkey and break it while cooking, cook for 5 minutes.

5. Add remaining ingredients and bring the mix to simmer.

6. Simmer for 15 minutes over low heat (lid off).

7. Pour chicken broth.

8. Serve with desired salad.

9. Enjoy!

Nutrition

- Calories: 312
- Fat: 16 g.
- Carbohydrates: 14 g.
- Protein: 27 g.

- Phosphorus: 196 mg.
- Potassium: 285 mg.
- Sodium: 171 mg.

5.13 ZUCCHINI ZOODLES WITH CHICKEN AND BASIL

Preparation time: 10 minutes - Cooking time: 10 minutes - Servings: 2

Ingredients

- 2 chicken fillets, cubed
- 2 tbsps. ghee
- 1 lb. tomatoes, diced
- ½ c. basil, chopped

- ¼ c. coconut almond milk
- 1 garlic clove, peeled, minced
- 1 zucchini, shredded
- Some Sunflower seeds

Directions

1. Sauté cubed chicken in ghee until no longer pink.

2. Add tomatoes and season with sunflower seeds.

3. Simmer and reduce the liquid.

4. Prepare your zucchini zoodles by shredding zucchini in a food processor.

5. Add basil, garlic, coconut almond milk to chicken and cook for a few minutes.

6. Add half of the zucchini zoodles to a bowl and top with creamy tomato basil chicken.

7. Enjoy!

Nutrition

- Calories: 540
- Fat: 27 g.
- Carbohydrates: 13 g.
- Sodium: 128 mg.

- Protein: 59 g.
- Phosphorus: 236 mg.
- Potassium: 290 mg.

5.14 TASTY ROASTED BROCCOLI

Preparation time: 5 minutes - Cooking time: 20 minutes - Servings: 4

Ingredients

- 4 c. broccoli florets
- 1 tbsp. olive oil
- Sunflower seeds and pepper to taste

Directions

1. Preheat your oven to 400°F.
2. Add broccoli in a zip bag alongside oil and shake until coated.
3. Add seasoning and shake again.
4. Spread broccoli out on a baking sheet, bake for 20 minutes.
5. Let it cool and serve.
6. Enjoy!

Nutrition

- Calories: 62
- Fat: 4 g.
- Carbohydrates: 4 g.
- Protein: 4 g.
- Phosphorus: 267 mg.
- Potassium: 285 mg.
- Sodium: 134 mg.

5.15 ALMOND BREADED CHICKEN GOODNESS

Preparation time: 15 minutes - Cooking time: 15 minutes - Servings: 3

Ingredients

- 2 large chicken breasts, boneless and skinless
- ⅓ c. lemon juice
- 1 ½ c. seasoned almond meal
- 2 tbsps. coconut oil
- Lemon pepper, to taste
- Parsley for decoration

Directions

1. Slice chicken breast in half.
2. Pound out each half until ¼-inch thick.
3. Take a pan and place it over medium heat, add oil, and heat it up.
4. Dip each chicken breast slice into lemon juice and let it sit for 2 minutes.
5. Turn over, and let the other side sit for 2 minutes as well.
6. Transfer to almond meal and coat both sides.
7. Add coated chicken to the oil and fry for 4 minutes per side, making sure to sprinkle lemon pepper liberally.
8. Transfer to a paper-lined sheet and repeat until all chicken is fried.
9. Garnish with parsley and enjoy!

Nutrition

- Calories: 325
- Fat: 24 g.
- Carbohydrates: 3 g.

- Protein: 16 g.
- Phosphorus: 196 mg.
- Potassium: 285 mg.

5.16 SODIUM: 111 MG.SOUTH-WESTERN PORK CHOPS

Preparation time: 10 minutes - Cooking time: 15 minutes - Servings: 4

Ingredients

- Cooking spray as needed
- 4 oz. pork loin chop, boneless and fat-rimmed

- ⅓ c. salsa
- 2 tbsps. fresh lime juice
- ¼ c. fresh cilantro, chopped

Directions

1. Take a large-sized nonstick skillet and spray it with cooking spray.
2. Heat until hot over high heat.
3. Press the chops with your palm to flatten them slightly.
4. Add them to the skillet and cook for 1 minute for each side until they are nicely browned.
5. Lower the heat to medium-low.
6. Combine the salsa and lime juice.
7. Pour the mix over the chops.
8. Simmer uncovered for about 8 minutes until the chops are perfectly done.
9. If needed, sprinkle some cilantro on top.

Nutrition

- Calories: 184
- Fat: 4 g.
- Carbohydrates: 4 g.
- Sodium: 98 mg.

- Protein: 0.5 g.
- Phosphorus: 196 mg.
- Potassium: 285 mg.

5.17 ALMOND BUTTER PORK CHOPS

Preparation time: 5 minutes - Cooking time: 25 minutes - Servings: 2

Ingredients

- 1 tbsp. almond butter, divided
- 2 boneless pork chops
- Pepper to taste
- 1 tbsp. dried Italian seasoning, low-fat and low-sodium
- 1 tbsp. olive oil

Directions

1. Preheat your oven to 350°F.
2. Pat pork chops dry with a paper towel and place them in a baking dish.
3. Season with pepper, and Italian seasoning.
4. Drizzle olive oil over pork chops.
5. Top each chop with ½ tbsp. almond butter.
6. Bake for 25 minutes.
7. Transfer pork chops on 2 plates and top with almond butter juice.
8. Serve and enjoy!

Nutrition

- Calories: 333
- Fat: 23 g.
- Carbohydrates: 1 g.
- Protein: 31 g.
- Phosphorus: 296 mg.
- Potassium: 285 mg.
- Sodium: 123 mg.

5.18 CHICKEN SALSA

Preparation time: 4 minutes - Cooking time: 14 minutes - Servings: 1

Ingredients

- 2 chicken breasts
- 1 c. salsa
- 1 taco seasoning mix
- 1 c. plain Greek Yogurt
- ½ c. Ricotta/Cashew cheese, cubed

Directions

1. Take a skillet and place it over medium heat.
2. Add chicken breast, ½ c. of salsa, and taco seasoning.
3. Mix well and cook for 12–15 minutes until the chicken is done.
4. Take the chicken out and cube them.
5. Place the cubes on a toothpick and top with cheese.
6. Place yogurt and remaining salsa in cups and use as dips.
7. Enjoy!

Nutrition

- Calories: 359
- Fat: 14 g.
- Net carbohydrates: 14 g.
- Protein: 43 g.

- Phosphorus: 196 mg.
- Potassium: 285 mg.
- Sodium: 111 mg.

5.19 HEALTHY MEDITERRANEAN LAMB CHOPS

Preparation time: 10 minutes - Cooking time: 10 minutes - Servings: 4

Ingredients

- 4 lamb shoulder chops, 8 oz. each
- 2 tbsps. Dijon mustard
- 2 tbsps. Balsamic vinegar

- ½ c. olive oil
- 2 tbsps. shredded fresh basil
- ½ tsp Pepper to taste

Directions

1. Pat your lamb chop dry using a kitchen towel and arrange them on a shallow glass baking dish.
2. Take a bowl and whisk in Dijon mustard, balsamic vinegar, pepper and mix them well.
3. Whisk in the oil very slowly into the marinade until the mixture is smooth.
4. Stir in basil.
5. Pour the marinade over the lamb chops and stir to coat both sides well.
6. Cover the chops and allow them to marinate for 1–4 hours (chilled).
7. Take the chops out and leave them for 30 minutes to allow the temperature to reach a normal level.
8. Preheat your grill to medium heat and add oil to the grate.
9. Grill the lamb chops for 5–10 minutes per side until both sides are browned.
10. Once the center reads 145°F, the chops are ready, serve and enjoy!

Nutrition

- Calories: 521
- Fat: 45 g.
- Carbohydrates: 3.5 g.
- Sodium: 111 mg.

- Protein: 22 g.
- Phosphorus: 226 mg.
- Potassium: 295 mg.

5.20   AMAZING SESAME BREADSTICKS

Preparation time: 10 minutes - Cooking time: 20 minutes - Servings: 5

Ingredients

- 1 egg white
- 2 tbsps. almond flour
- 1 tsp. Himalayan pink sunflower seeds
- 1 tbsp. extra-virgin olive oil
- ½ tsp. sesame seeds

Directions

1. Preheat your oven to 320°F.
2. Line a baking sheet with parchment paper and keep it on the side.
3. Take a bowl and whisk in egg whites, add flour and half of sunflower seeds and olive oil.
4. Knead until you have a smooth dough.
5. Divide into 4 pieces and roll into breadsticks.
6. Place on prepared sheet and brush with olive oil, sprinkle sesame seeds and remaining sunflower seeds.
7. Bake for 20 minutes.
8. Serve and enjoy!

Nutrition

- Total carbohydrates: 1.1 g.
- Fiber: 1 g.
- Protein: 1.6 g.
- Fat: 5 g.
- Phosphorus: 196 mg.
- Potassium: 285 mg.
- Sodium: 111 mg.

CHAPTER 6 - SEAFOOD RECIPES

6.1   FAMILY HIT CURRY

Preparation time: 10 minutes - Cooking time: 21 minutes - Servings: 8

Ingredients

- 1 ½ tbsp. canola oil
- 1 finely chopped onion
- 1 tsp. minced fresh ginger
- 3 minced garlic cloves
- 1 tbsp. curry paste
- 2 c. fat-free plain Greek yogurt
- ¼ c. water

- 1 tsp. sugar
- 1 lb. cubed cod fillets
- 1 lb. peeled and deveined prawns
- 1 pinch of salt
- Freshly ground black pepper, to taste
- 2 tbsp. fresh lemon juice
- ¼ c. chopped fresh cilantro leaves

Directions

1. In a large pan, heat oil on medium heat. Add onion and sauté for about 4–5 minutes.
2. Add ginger, garlic, and curry paste and sauté for about 1 minute.
3. Stir in yogurt, water, and sugar and bring to a boil on high heat.
4. Reduce the heat to medium-low. Simmer for about 5 minutes.
5. Stir in seafood and cook for about 10 minutes or till desired thickness.
6. Stir in salt, black pepper, lemon juice, and cilantro and remove from heat.
7. Serve hot.

Nutrition

- Calories: 191
- Fat: 5.3 g.
- Carbohydrates: 5 g.
- Protein: 29.2 g.

- Fiber: 0 g.
- Potassium: 270 mg.
- Sodium: 199 mg.

6.2 HOMEMADE TUNA NICOISE

Preparation time: 5 minutes - Cooking time: 10 minutes - Servings: 2

Ingredients

- 1 egg
- ½ c. green beans
- ¼ sliced cucumber
- 1 lemon's juice
- 1 tsp. black pepper
- ¼ sliced red onion

- 1 tbsp. olive oil
- 1 tbsp. capers
- 4 oz. drained canned tuna
- 4 iceberg lettuce leaves
- 1 tsp. chopped fresh cilantro

Directions

1. Prepare the salad by washing and slicing the lettuce, cucumber, and onion.
2. Add to a salad bowl.
3. Mix 1 tbsp. of oil with lemon juice, cilantro, and capers for a salad dressing. Set aside.
4. Boil a pan of water on high heat, then lower to simmer and add the egg for 6 minutes. (Steam the green beans over the same pan in a steamer/colander for 6 minutes.)
5. Remove the egg and rinse under cold water.
6. Peel before slicing in half.
7. Mix the tuna, salad, and dressing in a salad bowl.
8. Toss to coat.
9. Top with the egg and serve with a sprinkle of black pepper.

Nutrition

- Calories: 199
- Protein: 19 g.
- Carbohydrates: 7 g.
- Fat: 8 g.

- Sodium: 466 mg.
- Potassium: 251 mg.
- Phosphorus: 211 mg.

6.3 CAJUN CRAB

Preparation time: 10 minutes - Cooking time: 10 minutes - Servings: 2

Ingredients

- 1 lemon, fresh and quartered
- 3 tbsps. Cajun seasoning

- 2 bay leaves
- 4 snow crab legs, precooked and defrosted

- Golden ghee

Directions

1. Fill a large pot with salted water about halfway.
2. Bring the water to a boil.
3. Squeeze lemon juice into a pot and toss in the remaining lemon quarters.
4. Add bay leaves and Cajun seasoning.
5. Then season for 1 minute.
6. Add crab legs and boil for 8 minutes (make sure to keep them submerged the whole time).
7. Melt ghee in the microwave and use it as a dipping sauce, enjoy!

Nutrition

- Calories: 643
- Fat: 51 g.
- Carbohydrates: 3 g.
- Protein: 41 g.

6.4   CREAMY CRAB SOUP

Preparation time: 10 minutes - Cooking time: 15–20 minutes - Servings: 7–8

Ingredients

- 1 tbsp. low-salt butter
- 1 c. white onion, chopped
- ½ lb. fresh crab meat
- 4 c. low-salt chicken broth
- 1 c. soy or vegetable cream
- 2 tbsp. cornstarch
- ⅛ tsp. dill
- Kosher pepper

Directions

1. Melt the butter in a large pan over medium heat.
2. Add the onion to the pot and sauté until transparent, for around 3 minutes.
3. Add the crab meat to the mix and cook for another couple of minutes.
4. Add the chicken broth to the pan mix and bring to a boil.
5. Mix the vegetable or soy cream with the cornstarch and whisk to combine well. Add to the soup and increase the heat to medium-high.
6. Add the dill and pepper and stir frequently until the soup comes to a boil.
7. Serve hot.

Nutrition

- Calories: 89
- Carbohydrate: 10 g.
- Protein: 7 g.
- Sodium: 228 mg.
- Fat: 3.7 g.
- Potassium: 237 mg.
- Phosphorus: 83 mg.
- Dietary fiber: 0.3 g.

6.5   SPICY LIME SHRIMP

Preparation time: 10 minutes - Cooking time: 5 minutes - Servings: 4–5

Ingredients

- 32 large shrimp, peeled and deveined
- ¼ c. lime juice
- 1 garlic clove, minced
- 1 green onion, sliced
- 3 tbsp. red bell pepper, diced
- 2 tbsp. fresh cilantro, chopped
- 1 tsp. jalapeño chili, minced
- ⅛ tsp. salt
- 1 big cucumber, sliced

Directions

1. To make your dressing, combine the lime juice, green onion, red bell pepper, jalapeño chili, cilantro, garlic, and oil or salt in a mixing bowl.
2. In a separate mixing bowl, add the shrimps with 3 tbsp. of the lime juice marinade. Cover and let in the fridge for 40 minutes.
3. Turn on your oven's broiler. Discard the shrimp from the lime marinade and broil for around 3–4 minutes in total or 2 minutes on each side.
4. Take off the heat and pour the remaining marinade on top.
5. Place over the cucumber slices and serve cold.

Nutrition

- Calories: 132
- Carbohydrates: 3 g.
- Protein: 12 g.
- Sodium: 149 mg.
- Potassium: 202 mg.
- Phosphorus: 128 mg.
- Dietary fiber: 0.6 g.
- Fat: 8 g

6.6   SEAFOOD CASSEROLE

Preparation time: 20 minutes - Cooking time: 45 minutes - Servings: 6

Ingredients

- 2 c. eggplant, peeled and diced into 1-inch pieces
- Butter, for greasing the baking sheet
- 1 tbsp. olive oil
- ½ sweet onion, chopped
- 1 tsp. minced garlic
- 1 stalk of celery, chopped
- ½ red bell pepper, boiled and chopped
- 3 tbsps. freshly squeezed lemon juice
- 1 tsp. hot sauce
- ¼ tsp. creole seasoning mix
- ½ c. uncooked white rice
- 1 large egg
- 4 oz. cooked shrimp
- 6 oz. queen crab meat

Directions

1. Preheat the oven to 350°F.
2. Boil the eggplant in a saucepan for 5 minutes. Drain and set aside.

3. Grease a 9x13-inch baking sheet with butter and set aside.

4. Heat the olive oil in a large skillet over medium heat.

5. Sauté the garlic, onion, celery, and bell pepper for 4 minutes or until tender.

6. Add the sautéed vegetables to the eggplant, along with the lemon juice, hot sauce, seasoning, rice, and egg.

7. Stir to combine.

8. Fold in the shrimp and crab meat.

9. Spoon the casserole mixture into the casserole dish, patting down the top.

10. Bake for 25–30 minutes or until casserole is heated through and rice is tender.

11. Serve warm.

Nutrition

- Calories: 118
- Fat: 4 g.
- Carbohydrates: 9 g.
- Phosphorus: 102 mg.
- Potassium: 199 mg.
- Sodium: 235 mg.
- Protein: 12 g.

6.7   TILAPIA CEVICHE

Preparation time: 15 minutes - Cooking time: 5 minutes - Servings: 1

Ingredients

- 1 ½ lbs. fresh tilapia fillets
- 1 c. red onion
- ½ c. red bell pepper
- ¼ c. cilantro
- 1 c. pineapple
- 2 tbsps. canola oil
- ¼ tsp. black pepper
- 1 ¼ c. fresh lime juice
- 48 saltine crackers with unsalted tops

Directions

1. Chop the onion, bell pepper, and cilantro. Also, dice the pineapple, and cube the tilapia into small chunks.

2. Broil tilapia cubes over high heat for about 3 minutes on each side.

3. Cool the tilapia for about 5 minutes, then pour the fresh lime juice on top of it, mixing properly. Ensure all tilapia pieces are coated completely with the lime juice.

4. Combine and mix the bell pepper, onion, pineapple, cilantro, black pepper, and canola oil with the broiled tilapia mixture.

5. Cover and refrigerate to marinate for about 2 hours.

6. Use 6 saltine crackers with unsalted tops for each serving.

Nutrition

- Calories: 220
- Protein: 19 g.
- Carbohydrates: 20 g.
- Fat: 7 g.
- Cholesterol: 36 mg.
- Sodium: 168 mg.

- Potassium: 374 mg.
- Phosphorus: 162 mg.

- Fiber: 1.3 g.

6.8   FISH TACOS

Preparation time: 10 minutes - Cooking time: 35 minutes - Servings: 6

Ingredients

- 1 ½ c. cabbage
- ½ c. red onion
- ½ bunch of cilantro
- 1 garlic clove
- 2 limes
- 1 lb. cod fillets
- ½ tsp. ground cumin

- ½ tsp. chili powder
- ¼ tsp. black pepper
- 1 tbsp. olive oil
- ½ c. mayonnaise
- ¼ c. sour cream
- 2 tbsps. milk
- 12 (6-inch) corn tortillas

Directions

1. Shred the cabbage, chop the onion and cilantro, and mince the garlic. Set aside.
2. Use a dish to place in the fish fillets, then squeeze half a lime juice over the fish. Sprinkle the fish fillets with minced garlic, cumin, black pepper, chili powder, and olive oil. Turn the fish fillets to coat with the marinade, then refrigerate for about 15–30 minutes.
3. Prepare Salsa Blanca by mixing the mayonnaise, milk, sour cream, and the other half of the lime juice. Stir to combine, then place in the refrigerator to chill.
4. Broil in the oven and cover the broiler pan with aluminum foil. Broil the coated fish fillets for about 10 minutes or until the flesh becomes opaque and white and flakes easily. Remove from the oven, slightly cool, and then flake the fish into bigger pieces.
5. Heat the corn tortillas in a pan, one at a time until it becomes soft and warm, then wrap in a dish towel to keep them warm.
6. To assemble the tacos, place a piece of the fish on the tortilla, topping with the Salsa Blanca, cabbage, cilantro, red onion, and lime wedges.
7. Serve with hot sauce if you desire.

Nutrition

- Calories: 363
- Protein: 18 g.
- Carbohydrates: 30 g.
- Fat: 19 g.
- Fiber: 4.3 g.

- Cholesterol: 40 mg.
- Sodium: 194 mg.
- Potassium: 507 mg.
- Phosphorus: 327 mg.

6.9 JAMBALAYA

Preparation time: 10 minutes - Cooking time: 1 hour and 15 minutes - Servings: 12

Ingredients

- 2 c. onion
- 1 c. bell pepper
- 2 garlic cloves
- 2 c. uncooked converted brown rice
- ½ tsp. black pepper
- 8 oz. canned low-sodium tomato sauce
- 2 c. low-sodium beef broth
- 2 lbs. raw shrimp
- ½ c. unsalted margarine

Directions

1. Preheat oven to 350°F.
2. Chop the onion, bell pepper, garlic, then peel the shrimp.
3. Combine and mix all the ingredients in a large bowl except the margarine.
4. Pour into a 9x13-inch baking sheet and evenly spread out.
5. Slice the margarine, placing it over the top of the ingredients.
6. Cover with foil or lid, and bake for about 1 hour and 15 minutes.
7. Serve hot.

Nutrition

- Calories: 294
- Protein: 20 g.
- Carbohydrates: 31 g.
- Fat: 10 g.
- Cholesterol: 137 mg.
- Sodium: 186 mg.
- Potassium: 300 mg.
- Phosphorus: 197 mg.
- Fiber: 0.8 g.

6.10 ASPARAGUS SHRIMP LINGUINI

Preparation time: 10 minutes - Cooking time: 35 minutes - Servings: 1 ½

Ingredients

- 8 oz. uncooked linguini
- 2 tbsps. olive oil
- 1 ¾ c. asparagus
- ½ c. unsalted butter
- 2 garlic cloves
- 3 oz. cream cheese
- 2 tbsps. fresh parsley
- ¾ tsp. dried basil
- ⅔ c. dry white wine
- ½ lb. peeled and cooked shrimp

Directions

1. Preheat oven to 350°F.
2. Cook the linguini in boiling water until it becomes tender, then drain.
3. Place the asparagus on a baking sheet, then spread 2 tbsps. of oil over the asparagus. Bake for about 7–8 minutes or until it is tender.
4. Remove baked asparagus from the oven and place it on a plate. Cut the asparagus into pieces of medium-sized once cooled.

5. Mince the garlic and chop the parsley.

6. Melt ½ c. of butter in a large skillet with minced garlic.

7. Stir in the cream cheese, mixing as it melts.

8. Stir in the parsley and basil, then simmer for about 5 minutes. Mix either in boiling water or dry white wine, stirring until the sauce becomes smooth.

9. Add the cooked shrimp and asparagus, then stir and heat until it is evenly warm.

10. Toss the cooked pasta with the sauce and serve.

Nutrition

- Calories: 544
- Protein: 21 g.
- Carbohydrates: 43 g.
- Fat: 32 g.
- Cholesterol: 188 mg.

- Sodium: 170 mg.
- Potassium: 402 mg.
- Phosphorus: 225 mg.
- Fiber: 2.4 g.

6.11 TUNA NOODLE CASSEROLE

Preparation time: 10 minutes - Cooking time: 30 minutes - Servings: 2

Ingredients

- 2 oz. wide uncooked egg noodles
- 5 oz. canned tuna in water
- ½ c. sour cream
- ¼ c. cottage cheese

- ½ c. fresh sliced mushrooms
- ½ c. frozen green peas
- 1 tbsp. unsalted butter
- ¼ c. unseasoned breadcrumbs

Directions

1. Preheat oven to 350°F.

2. Boil egg noodles based on the package instructions and drain. Also, drain and flake the tuna.

3. Combine and mix the sour cream, cottage cheese, mushrooms, tuna, and peas in a medium bowl.

4. Stir the drained noodle into the tuna mixture, and place it in a small casserole dish that has been sprayed with a nonstick cooking spray.

5. Melt butter, stir into the breadcrumbs, then sprinkle over the mixture of noodles in step 4.

6. Bake for about 20–25 minutes or until the breadcrumbs start to brown.

7. Divide into 2 and serve.

Nutrition

- Calories: 415
- Protein: 22 g.
- Carbohydrates: 39 g.
- Fat: 19 g.
- Cholesterol: 88 mg.
- Sodium: 266 mg.
- Potassium: 400 mg.

- Phosphorus: 306 mg.
- Fiber: 3.2 g.

6.12 OVEN-FRIED SOUTHERN STYLE CATFISH

Preparation time: 10 minutes - Cooking time: 25 minutes - Servings: 4

Ingredients

- 1 egg white
- ½ c. all-purpose flour
- ¼ c. cornmeal
- ¼ c. panko breadcrumbs
- 1 tsp. salt-free Cajun seasoning
- 1 lb. catfish fillets

Directions

8. Heat oven to 450°F.
9. Use cooking spray to spray a nonstick baking sheet.
10. Using a bowl, beat the egg white until very soft peaks are formed. Don't over-beat.
11. Use a sheet of wax paper and place the flour over it.
12. Use a different sheet of wax paper to combine and mix the cornmeal, panko, and Cajun seasoning.
13. Cut the catfish fillet into 4 pieces, then dip the fish in the flour, shaking off the excess.
14. Dip coated fish in the egg white, rolling into the cornmeal mixture.
15. Place the fish on the baking pan. Repeat with the remaining fish fillets.
16. Use cooking spray to spray over the fish fillets. Bake for about 10–12 minutes or until the sides of the fillets become browned and crisp.

Nutrition

- Calories: 250
- Protein: 22 g.
- Carbohydrates: 19 g.
- Fat: 10 g.
- Cholesterol: 53 mg.
- Sodium: 124 mg.
- Potassium: 401 mg.
- Phosphorus: 262 mg.

6.13 FIBER: 1.2 G. CILANTRO-LIME COD

Preparation time: 10 minutes - Cooking time: 20 minutes - Servings: 4

Ingredients

- ½ c. mayonnaise
- ½ c. fresh chopped cilantro
- 2 tbsp. lime juice
- 1 lb. cod fillets

Directions

1. Combine and mix the mayonnaise, cilantro, and lime juice in a medium bowl, remove ¼ c. to another bowl and put aside. To be served as fish sauce.
2. Spread the remaining mayonnaise mixture over the cod fillets.
3. Use cooking spray to spray a large skillet, then heat over medium-high heat.
4. Place in the cod fillets, and cook for about 8 minutes or until the fish becomes firm and moist, turning just once.
5. Serve with the ¼ cilantro-lime sauce.

Nutrition

- Calories: 292
- Protein: 20 g.
- Carbohydrates: 1 g.
- Fat: 23 g.
- Cholesterol: 57 mg.

- Sodium: 228 mg.
- Potassium: 237 mg.
- Phosphorus: 128 mg.
- Calcium: 14 mg.

6.14 CITRUS GRILLED GLAZED SALMON

Preparation time: 10 minutes . Cooking time: 20 minutes - Servings: 6

Ingredients

- 2 garlic cloves
- 1 ½ tbsps. lemon juice
- 2 tbsps. olive oil
- 1 tbsp. unsalted butter
- 1 tbsp. Dijon mustard

- 2 dashes of cayenne pepper
- 1 tsp. dried basil leaves
- 1 tsp. dried dill
- 1 tbsp. capers
- 24 oz. salmon fillet

Directions

1. Crush the garlic.
2. Combine all ingredients in a small saucepan, excluding the salmon, heat to a boil, then reduce the heat to low, cook for about 5 minutes.
3. Preheat grill, then place the salmon with its skin side down on a sheet of foil that is a little bigger than the fish. Fold up the edges so that the sauce remains with the salmon on the grill. Place on top of the grill, the foil, and fish, then top the salmon with the sauce mixture from step 2.
4. Cover grill and cook for about 12 minutes or until the salmon has cooked (don't flip the salmon).
5. Cut the salmon into 6 servings.

Nutrition

- Calories: 294
- Protein: 23 g.
- Carbohydrates: 1 g.
- Fat: 22 g.
- Cholesterol: 68 mg.

- Sodium: 190 mg.
- Potassium: 439 mg.
- Phosphorus: 280 mg.
- Fiber: 0.2 g.

6.15 OMEGA-3 RICH SALMON

Preparation time: 10 minutes - Cooking time: 20–25 minutes - Servings: 2

Ingredients

- 2 (4 oz.) skinless, boneless salmon fillets
- 2 tbsp. fresh lemon juice
- 1 tbsp. olive oil

- ¼ tsp. crushed dried oregano
- 1 pinch of salt
- Freshly ground black pepper, to taste

Directions

1. Preheat the oven to 425°F. Line a baking sheet with parchment paper.
2. Place the salmon fillets onto the prepared baking sheet.
3. Drizzle with lemon juice and oil evenly and sprinkle with oregano, salt, and black pepper.
4. Bake for about 20–25 minutes.
5. Serve hot.

Nutrition

- Calories: 265
- Fat: 19.2 g.
- Carbohydrates: 0.5 g.
- Protein: 22.3 g.
- Fiber: 0 g.
- Potassium: 23 mg.
- Sodium: 146 mg.

6.16 WHOLESOME SALMON MEAL

Preparation time: 10 minutes - Cooking time: 20–25 minutes - Servings: 6

Ingredients

- 4 (6 oz.) (1-inch thick) skinless salmon fillets
- Freshly ground black pepper, to taste
- 2 c. finely chopped zucchini, chopped finely
- 1 c. halved cherry tomatoes
- 1 tbsp. olive oil
- 1 tbsp. fresh lemon juice

Directions

1. Preheat the oven to 425°F. Grease an 11x7-inch baking sheet.
2. Place the salmon fillets in the prepared baking sheet in a single layer and sprinkle with black pepper generously.
3. In a bowl, mix the remaining ingredients.
4. Place the mixture over salmon fillets evenly.
5. Bake for about 22 minutes.
6. Remove from the oven and keep aside to cool slightly.
7. Cut the salmon into small chunks and mix with the veggie mixture.
8. Serve warm.

Nutrition

- Calories: 233
- Fat: 14.5 g.
- Carbohydrates: 2.5 g.
- Sodium: 71 mg.
- Protein: 22.9 g.
- Fiber: 0.8 g.
- Potassium: 173 mg.

6.17 SUCCULENT TILAPIA

Preparation time: 10 minutes - Cooking time: 12–15 minutes - Servings: 4

Ingredients

- 2 tbsp. unsalted margarine
- 4 minced garlic cloves
- 1 tsp. chopped fresh parsley
- Freshly ground black pepper, to taste
- 1 pinch of Mrs. Dash salt-free herb seasoning
- 4 (4 oz.) tilapia fillets

Directions

1. Preheat the oven to 350°F. Line a shallow baking sheet with a piece of foil.
2. In a large nonstick skillet, add margarine, garlic, parsley, black pepper, and seasoning on low heat.
3. Cook till melted completely, stirring continuously.
4. Remove from heat.
5. At the bottom of a prepared baking sheet, spread a little of the garlic sauce evenly.
6. Arrange the tilapia fillets over the garlic sauce.
7. Coat the top of each tilapia fillet with the garlic sauce evenly.
8. Bake for about 12–15 minutes.

Nutrition

- Calories: 149
- Fat: 6.7 g.
- Carbohydrates: 1.1 g.
- Protein: 21.4 g.
- Fiber: 0 g.
- Potassium: 17 mg.
- Sodium: 107 mg.

6.18 FESTIVE TILAPIA

Preparation time: 10 minutes - Cooking time: 3 minutes - Servings: 8

Ingredients

- ⅓ c. shredded low-fat Parmesan cheese
- 2 tbsp. low-sodium mayonnaise
- ¼ c. softened unsalted butter
- 2 tbsp. fresh lemon juice
- 2 lbs. tilapia fillets
- ¼ tsp. crushed dried thyme
- Freshly ground black pepper, to taste

Directions

1. Preheat the broiler. Grease the broiler pan.
2. In a large bowl, mix all ingredients except tilapia fillets. Keep aside.
3. Place the fillets onto the prepared broiler pan in a single layer.
4. Broil the fillets for about 2–3 minutes.
5. Remove from the oven and top the fillets with cheese mixture evenly.
6. Broil for about 2 minutes more.

Nutrition

- Calories: 176
- Fat: 9.1 g.
- Carbohydrates: 1.2 g.
- Protein: 22.9 g.
- Fiber: 0 g.
- Potassium: 7 mg.
- Sodium: 156 mg.

6.19 SALMON STUFFED PASTA

Preparation time: 20 minutes - Cooking time: 35 minutes - Servings: 24

Ingredients

- 24 jumbo pasta shells, boiled
- 1 c. coffee creamer

For the filling:

- 2 eggs, beaten
- 2 c. creamed cottage cheese
- ¼ c. chopped onion
- 1 red bell pepper, diced
- 2 tsps. dried parsley
- ½ tsp. lemon peel
- 1 can salmon, drained

For the dill sauce:

- 1 ½ tsp. butter
- 1 ½ tsp. flour
- ⅛ tsp. pepper
- 1 tbsp. lemon juice
- 1 ½ c. coffee creamer
- 2 tsps. dried dill weed

Directions

1. Beat the egg with the cream cheese and all the other filling ingredients in a bowl.
2. Divide the filling in the pasta shells and place the shells in a 9x13-inch baking dish.
3. Pour the coffee creamer around the stuffed shells then cover with a foil.
4. Bake the shells for 30 minutes at 350°F.
5. Meanwhile, whisk all the ingredients for dill sauce in a saucepan.
6. Stir for 5 minutes until it thickens.
7. Pour this sauce over the baked pasta shells.
8. Serve warm.

Nutrition

- Calories: 268
- Total fat: 4.8 g.
- Sodium: 86 mg.
- Potassium: 181 mg.
- Protein: 11.5 g.
- Calcium: 27 mg.
- Phosphorus: 314 mg.

6.20 HERBED VEGETABLE TROUT

Preparation time: 15 minutes - Cooking time: 15 minutes - Servings: 4

Ingredients

- 14 oz. trout fillets
- ½ tsp. herb seasoning blend
- 1 lemon, sliced
- 2 green onions, sliced
- 1 stalk celery, chopped
- 1 medium carrot, julienne

Directions

1. Prepare and preheat a charcoal grill over moderate heat.
2. Place the trout fillets over a large piece of foil and drizzle herb seasoning on top.
3. Spread the lemon slices, carrot, celery, and green onions over the fish.
4. Cover the fish with foil and pack it.
5. Place the packed fish in the grill and cook for 15 minutes.
6. Once done, remove the foil from the fish.
7. Serve.

Nutrition

- Calories: 202
- Total fat: 8.5 g.
- Sodium: 82 mg.
- Calcium: 70 mg.
- Phosphorus: 287 mg.
- Potassium: 560 mg.

CHAPTER 7 - POULTRY AND MEAT RECIPES

7.1   CURRIED CHICKEN STIR-FRY

Preparation time: 20 minutes - Cooking time: 15 minutes - Servings: 6

Ingredients

- 12 oz. chicken breasts, 1-inch cubes, boneless skinless
- 2 tsps. curry powder
- ⅛ tsp. salt
- ⅛ tsp. freshly ground black pepper
- 1 (20 oz.) can of pineapple tidbits, strained, reserving juice
- 2 tbsps. extra-virgin olive oil
- 1 yellow onion, chopped
- 2 red bell peppers, chopped

Directions

1. In a medium bowl, toss the chicken, curry powder, salt, and pepper and set aside.

2. In a small saucepan, heat the reserved pineapple juice over low heat. Let it reduce, occasionally stirring, while you make the rest of the stir-fry.

3. Heat the large skillet with olive oil in medium heat. Add the chicken. Stir-fry for 3 for 4 minutes or until the chicken is light brown; it doesn't have to completely cook. Transfer the chicken to a plate.

4. Put the onion into the skillet and cook for 3 minutes, stirring, until the onion is crisp-tender. Check to make sure the pineapple liquid isn't burning and continue to stir it. Add bell peppers then stir-fry it for another 3 minutes, until crisp-tender.

5. Put the chicken back to the skillet, add the pineapple tidbits and cook, stirring, for 3–4 minutes or until the chicken is cooked through.

6. Add the thickened pineapple juice to the skillet and stir.

7. Serve.

Nutrition

- Calories: 215
- Total fat: 7 g.
- Saturated fat: 1 g.
- Sodium: 98 mg.
- Phosphorus: 146 mg.
- Potassium: 374 mg.
- Carbohydrates: 19 g.
- Fiber: 2 g.
- Protein: 19 g.
- Sugar: 16 g.

7.2   THAI-STYLE CHICKEN SALAD

Preparation time: 10 minutes - Cooking time: 20 minutes - Servings: 6

Ingredients

- 3 c. (1 lb.) cooked chicken, shredded
- 1 (10 oz.) package shredded cabbage with carrots
- 2 limes
- ⅓ c. extra-virgin olive oil
- ¼ c. peanut butter
- ¼ tsp. freshly ground black pepper
- ¼ c. chopped peanuts

Directions

1. Combine the chicken and cabbage with carrots and toss to mix in a large bowl.
2. In a small bowl, zest one of the limes. Juice both of the limes into the bowl. Add the olive oil, peanut butter, and pepper and mix with a whisk.
3. Drizzle the dressing over the salad and toss. Top with the peanuts and serve.
4. Ingredient tip: If you like spicy food, add 1–2 minced jalapeño peppers to this salad. You could also add minced chipotle peppers in adobo sauce; just 1 tsp. of each will add lots of heat.

Nutrition

- Calories: 415
- Total fat: 31 g.
- Saturated fat: 5 g.
- Sodium: 119 mg.
- Phosphorus: 239 mg.
- Potassium: 408 mg.
- Carbohydrates: 9 g.
- Fiber: 3 g.
- Protein: 28 g.
- Sugar: 3 g.

7.3   FLAVORFUL PORK CHOP

Preparation time: 6 minutes - Cooking time: 14 minutes - Servings: 4

Ingredients

- ¼ c. of minced fresh basil
- 2 minced garlic cloves
- 2 tbsp. of olive oil
- 2 tbsp. of fresh lemon juice
- 1 pinch of salt
- Freshly ground black pepper, to taste
- 4 bone-in pork loin chops

Directions

1. In a large bowl, mix all ingredients except chops.
2. Add chops and coat with mixture generously.
3. Cover and keep aside to marinate for about 30–45 minutes.
4. Preheat the grill to medium-high heat. Grease the grill grate.
5. Grill for about 6 minutes per side.

Nutrition

- Calories: 267
- Fat: 13.5 g.
- Carbohydrates: 0.9 g.
- Protein: 35.9 g.
- Fiber: 0 g.
- Potassium: 20 mg.
- Sodium: 41 mg.

7.4   CREAMY CHICKEN

Preparation time: 10 minutes - Cooking time: 15 minutes - Servings: 2

Ingredients

- 3 tbsps. unsalted butter
- 2 lbs. cut into 1-inch-thick strips skinless, boneless chicken breasts
- 4 minced garlic cloves
- ½ tsp. ground ginger
- ½ tsp. ground coriander
- ½ tsp. ground cumin
- ¼ tsp. crushed red pepper flakes
- ½ c. chicken broth
- ⅓ c. low-fat sour cream
- 1 tbsp. chopped fresh parsley

Directions

1. In a large skillet, melt butter on medium-high heat.
2. Add chicken and cook for about 5–6 minutes.
3. Add garlic and spices and cook for 1 minute.
4. Add broth and bring to a boil. Reduce the heat to medium-low.
5. Simmer for about 5 minutes, stirring occasionally.
6. Stir in cream and simmer, occasionally stirring for about 3 minutes.
7. Serve hot with the garnishing of parsley.

Nutrition

- Calories: 206
- Fat: 10.5 g.
- Carbohydrates: 1.2 g.
- Sodium: 144 mg.
- Protein: 26.1 g.
- Fiber: 0 g.
- Potassium: 43 mg.

7.5   FABULOUS CHICKEN

Preparation time: 10 minutes - Cooking time: 15 minutes - Servings: 8

Ingredients

- 1 c. low-sodium chicken broth
- 3 tbsp. balsamic vinegar
- 2 tsp. cornstarch
- 2 tbsp. olive oil
- 4 minced garlic cloves
- 2 tbsp. minced fresh basil
- 4 (4 oz.) skinless, boneless chicken breasts
- 1 pinch of salt
- Freshly ground black pepper, to taste
- 2 cored and sliced pears

Directions

1. In a bowl, mix broth, vinegar, and cornstarch.
2. In a large skillet, heat oil on medium-high heat.
3. Add garlic and basil and sauté for about 1 minute.
4. Add chicken and sprinkle with salt and black pepper.
5. Cook for about 12–15 minutes. Transfer the chicken into a bowl.
6. In the same skillet, add pears and cook for about 4–5 minutes.
7. Add broth mixture and bring to a boil, cook for about 1 minute.
8. Reduce the heat to low.
9. Stir in chicken and cook for about 3–4 minutes.

Nutrition

- Calories: 279
- Fat: 11.2 g.
- Carbohydrates: 18.8 g.
- Protein: 26.4 g.
- Fiber: 3.8 g.
- Potassium: 145 mg.
- Sodium: 60 mg.

7.6   DIVINE GROUND CHICKEN

Preparation time: 10 minutes - Cooking time: 21 minutes - Servings: 5

Ingredients

- 1 ¼ lb. lean ground chicken
- 1 small sliced onion
- 2 tsp. minced garlic
- 1 tsp. ground cumin
- 1 tsp. ground coriander
- ⅛ tsp. ground turmeric
- ⅛ tsp. cayenne pepper
- 1 pinch of salt
- Freshly ground black pepper
- 1 chopped medium tomato
- 1 c. water
- ¼ c. chopped fresh cilantro, chopped

Directions

1. Heat a nonstick skillet on medium-high heat.
2. Add chicken, onion, and garlic and cook for about 5–6 minutes or till browned.
3. Remove any excess fat from the skillet.

4. Add spices and tomato cook for about 2 minutes.
5. Stir in water and bring to a gentle boil.
6. Reduce the heat to medium-low and simmer, covered for about 10–15 minutes.
7. Stir in cilantro and serve immediately.

Nutrition

- Calories: 164
- Fat: 6.2 g.
- Carbohydrates: 2.9 g.
- Protein: 23.5 g.

- Fiber: 0.7 g.
- Potassium: 161 mg.
- Sodium: 99 mg.

7.7   COMFORTING CHICKEN CHILI

Preparation time: 10 minutes - Cooking time: 2 hours - Servings: 12

Ingredients

- 2 tbsp. olive oil
- 1 chopped large onion
- 1 seeded and chopped medium green bell pepper
- 1 seeded and chopped medium red bell pepper
- 4 minced garlic cloves
- 1 chopped jalapeño pepper
- 1 tsp. crushed dried basil

- 1 tsp. crushed dried thyme
- 1 tbsp. red chili powder
- 1 tbsp. ground cumin
- 2 lbs. lean ground chicken
- 8 oz. low-sodium tomato paste
- 2 c. low-sodium chicken broth
- 2 c. water
- ½ tbsp. Ground black pepper to taste

Directions

1. In a large pan, heat oil on medium heat.
2. Add onion and bell pepper and sauté for about 5–7 minutes.
3. Add garlic, jalapeño pepper, herbs, spices, and black pepper and sauté for about 1 minute.
4. Add chicken and cook for about 4–5 minutes.
5. Stir in tomato paste and cook for about 2 minutes.
6. Add broth and water and bring to a boil.
7. Reduce the heat to low and simmer, covered for about 1–1 ½ hours or till the desired doneness.
8. Serve hot.

Nutrition

- Calories: 155
- Fat: 6.7 g.
- Carbohydrates: 7.4 g.
- Sodium: 123 mg.

- Protein: 17.1 g.
- Fiber: 1.6 g.
- Potassium: 275 mg.

7.8   SIMPLE LAMB CHOPS

Preparation time: 35 minutes - Cooking time: 5 minutes - Servings: 3

Ingredients

- ¼ c. olive oil
- ¼ c. mint, fresh and chopped
- 8 lamb rib chops
- 1 tbsp. garlic, minced
- 1 tbsp. rosemary, fresh and chopped

Directions

1. Add rosemary, garlic, mint, olive oil into a bowl and mix well.
2. Keep 1 tbsp. of the mixture on the side for later use.
3. Toss lamb chops into the marinade, letting them marinate for 30 minutes.
4. Take a cast-iron skillet and place it over medium-high heat.
5. Add lamb and cook for 2 minutes per side for medium-rare.
6. Let the lamb rest for a few minutes and drizzle the remaining marinade.
7. Serve and enjoy!

Nutrition

- Calories: 566
- Fat: 40 g.
- Carbohydrates: 2 g.
- Protein: 47 g.

7.9   BEER PORK RIBS

Preparation time: 35 minutes - Cooking time: 8 hours - Servings: 6

Ingredients

- 2 lbs. pork ribs, cut in 2 units/racks
- 18 oz. root beer
- 2 cloves of garlic, minced
- 2 tbsps. onion powder
- 2 tbsps. vegetable oil (optional)

Directions

1. Wrap the pork ribs with vegetable oil and place 1 unit on the bottom of your Slow Cooker with half of the minced garlic and the onion powder. Place the other rack on top with the rest of the garlic and onion powder.
2. Pour over the root beer and cover the lid.
3. Let simmer for 8 hours on low heat.
4. Take off and finish optionally in a grilling pan for a nice sear.

Nutrition

- Calories: 301
- Carbohydrates: 36 g.
- Protein: 21 g.
- Sodium: 729 mg.
- Potassium: 200 mg.
- Phosphorus: 209 mg.
- Dietary fiber: 0 g.
- Fat: 18 g.

7.10 MEXICAN STEAK TACOS

Preparation time: 10 minutes - Cooking time: 15 minutes - Servings: 8

Ingredients

- 1 lb. flank or skirt steak
- ¼ c. fresh cilantro, chopped
- ¼ c. white onion, chopped
- 3 limes, juiced
- 3 cloves of garlic, minced
- 2 tsp. garlic powder
- 2 tbsps. olive oil
- ½ c. Mexican or mozzarella cheese, grated
- 1 tsp. Mexican seasoning
- 8 medium-sized (6-inch) corn flour tortillas

Directions

1. Combine the juice from 2 limes, Mexican seasoning, and garlic powder in a dish or bowl, and marinate the steak with it for at least ½ hour in the fridge.
2. In a separate bowl, combine the chopped cilantro, garlic, onion, and juice from one lime to make your salsa. Cover and keep in the fridge.
3. Heat the olive oil in a medium pan. Slice steak into thin strips and cook for approx. 3 minutes on each side.
4. Preheat your oven to 350°F/180°C.
5. Distribute the steak strips evenly in each tortilla. Top with 1 tbsp. of grated cheese on top.
6. Wrap each taco in aluminum foil and bake in the oven for approx. 7–8 minutes or until cheese is melted.
7. Serve warm with your cilantro salsa.

Nutrition

- Calories: 230
- Carbohydrates: 19.5 g.
- Protein: 15 g.
- Sodium: 486.75 g.
- Fat: 11 g.
- Potassium: 240 mg.
- Phosphorus: 268 mg.
- Dietary fiber: 0.1 g.

7.11   MEXICAN CHORIZO SAUSAGE

Preparation time: 15 minutes - Cooking time: 15 minutes - Servings: 16

Ingredients

- 2 lbs. boneless pork but, coarsely ground
- 3 tbsps. red wine vinegar
- 2 tbsps. smoked paprika
- ½ tsp. cinnamon
- ½ tsp. ground cloves
- ¼ tsp. coriander seeds
- ¼ tsp. ground ginger
- 1 tsp. ground cumin
- 3 tbsps. brandy

Directions

1. In a large mixing bowl, combine the ground pork with the seasonings, brandy, and vinegar and mix with your hands well.
2. Place the mixture into a large Ziplock bag and leave it in the fridge overnight, for all the flavors to blend with each other and for lightly curing the sausage.
3. Form into 15–16 patties of equal size.
4. Heat the oil in a large pan and fry the patties for approx. 5–7 minutes on each side, or until the meat inside is no longer pink and there is a light brown crust on top.
5. Serve hot.

Nutrition

- Calories: 134
- Carbohydrates: 0 g.
- Protein: 10 g.
- Sodium: 40 mg.
- Potassium: 138 mg.
- Phosphorus: 128 mg.
- Dietary fiber: 0 g.
- Fat: 7 g.

7.12   CARIBBEAN TURKEY CURRY

Preparation time: 10 minutes - Cooking time: 1 hour 30 minutes - Servings: 6

Ingredients

- 3 ½ lb. turkey breast, with skin
- ¼ c. butter, melted
- ¼ c. honey
- 1 tbsp. mustard
- 2 tsp. curry powder
- 1 tsp. garlic powder

Directions

1. Place the turkey breast in a shallow roasting pan.
2. Insert a meat thermometer to monitor the temperature.
3. Bake the turkey for 1 ½ hours at 350°F until its internal temperature (as read by a meat thermometer) reaches 170°F.
4. Meanwhile, thoroughly mix honey, butter, curry powder, garlic powder, and mustard in a bowl.
5. Glaze the cooked turkey with this mixture liberally.
6. Let it sit for 15 minutes for absorption.
7. Slice and serve.

Nutrition

- Calories: 275
- Protein: 26 g.
- Carbohydrates: 9 g.
- Fat: 13 g.
- Cholesterol: 82 mg.

- Sodium: 122 mg.
- Potassium: 277 mg.
- Phosphorus: 193 mg.
- Calcium: 24 mg.
- Fiber: 0.2 g.

7.13 LEMON AND FRUIT PORK KEBABS

Preparation time: 20 minutes - Cooking time: 10 minutes - Servings: 4

Ingredients

- 8 oz. boneless pork loin chops, cubed
- 1 c. canned pineapple chunks, drained, reserving ¼ c. juice
- 2 peaches, peeled and cubed
- 4 scallions, white and green parts, cut into 2-inch pieces

- 2 tbsps. olive oil
- 1 lemon juice
- 2 tbsps. mustard
- 1 tbsp. cornstarch
- 2 tsps. packed brown sugar

Directions

1. Prepare and preheat the grill to medium coals and set a grill 6-inch from the coals.
2. Thread the pork cubes, pineapple, peach cubes, and scallion pieces onto 4 (10-inch) metal skewers. Drizzle the kebabs with olive oil and set them aside.
3. In a small saucepan, stir together the reserved pineapple juice, lemon juice, mustard, cornstarch, and brown sugar and bring to a simmer over medium heat. Simmer for 2–3 minutes or until the sauce boils and thickens. Remove from heat.
4. Place the kebabs on the grill. Grill for 8–10 minutes, turning frequently and brushing with the sauce until the pork registers at least 145°F internal temperature. Use all of the sauce.
5. Remove the kebabs from the heat and let stand for 5 minutes before serving.
6. Pork can be cooked to medium-well and still be considered food safe. Cook it to at least 145°F, measured with a meat thermometer, and let the pork stand for 5 minutes. This waits time will raise the temperature to 150°F and maintain its juiciness.

Nutrition

- Calories: 273
- Total fat: 13 g.
- Saturated fat: 3 g.
- Sodium: 118 mg.
- Potassium: 471 mg.
- Sugar: 17 g.

- Phosphorus: 158 mg.
- Carbohydrates: 22 g.
- Fiber: 2 g.
- Protein: 18 g.

7.14 CHICKEN STEW

Preparation time: 20 minutes - Cooking time: 50 minutes - Servings: 6

Ingredients

- 1 tbsp. olive oil
- 1 lb. chicken thighs, boneless, skinless (1-inch cubes)
- ½ sweet onion, chopped
- 1 tbsp. minced garlic
- 2 c. chicken stock
- 1 c. water, plus 2 tbsp.
- 1 sliced carrot
- 2 stalks of celery, sliced
- 1 turnip, sliced thin
- 1 tbsp. chopped fresh thyme
- 1 tsp. chopped fresh rosemary
- 2 tsp. cornstarch
- Ground black pepper to taste

Directions

1. Place a large saucepan on medium heat and add the olive oil.
2. Sauté the chicken for 6 minutes or until it is lightly browned, stirring often.
3. Add the onion and garlic, and sauté for 3 minutes.
4. Add 1 c. of water, chicken stock, carrot, celery, and turnip and bring the stew to a boil.
5. Reduce the heat to low and simmer for 30 minutes or until the chicken is cooked through and tender.
6. Add the thyme and rosemary and simmer for 3 minutes more.
7. In a small bowl, stir together the 2 tbsp. of water and the cornstarch.
8. Add the mixture to the stew.
9. Stir to incorporate the cornstarch mixture and cook for 3–4 minutes or until the stew thickens.
10. Remove from the heat and season with pepper.

Nutrition

- Calories: 141
- Fat: 8 g.
- Carbohydrates: 5 g.
- Protein: 9 g.
- Phosphorus: 53 mg.
- Potassium: 192 mg.
- Sodium: 214 mg.

7.15 ASIAN STYLE PAN-FRIED CHICKEN

Preparation time: 10 minutes - Cooking time: 20 minutes - Servings: 4

Ingredients

- 1 lemon, cut into wedges
- 3 tsp. canola oil, divided
- ½ c. cornstarch
- 1 tsp. low-sodium soy sauce
- 1-inch piece of minced ginger
- 1 tsp. dry rice wine
- 12 oz. chicken thighs, boneless and skinless

Directions

1. Mix the soy sauce, ginger, rice wine, and chicken.
2. Toss everything together and allow it to marinate for 15 minutes.
3. Toss the chicken one more time and then drain off the liquid. One at a time, dip the chicken pieces into the cornstarch so that they are coated.
4. Heat 1 ½ tsps. of oil on medium-high in a medium skillet.
5. Add half of the chicken to the skillet and cook until it has turned golden brown on one side, around 3–5 minutes. Turn the chicken over and continue to cook until the chicken has cooked through and browned. Place on a plate lined with a paper towel to cool and absorb excess oil.
6. Add in the remaining oil and cook the rest of the chicken thighs.
7. Serve the chicken with a garnish of lemon. Enjoy!

Nutrition

- Calories: 198
- Protein: 17 g.
- Sodium: 119 mg.
- Potassium: 218 mg.
- Phosphorus: 148 mg.

7.16 CURRIED CHICKEN WITH CAULIFLOWER

Preparation time: 20 minutes - Cooking time: 2 hours and 30 minutes - Servings: 6

Ingredients

- Lime juice of 2 limes
- ½ tsp. dried oregano
- Cauliflower head, cut into florets
- 4 tsp. extra-virgin olive oil, divided
- 6 chicken thighs, bone-in
- ½ tsp. pepper, divided
- ¼ tsp. paprika
- ½ tsp. ground cumin
- 3 tbsp. curry powder

Directions

1. Mix ¼ tsp. of pepper, paprika, cumin, and curry in a small bowl.
2. Add the chicken thighs to a medium bowl and drizzle with 2 tsp. of olive oil and sprinkle in the curry mixture.
3. Toss them together so that the chicken is well coated.
4. Cover this up and refrigerate it for at least 2 hours.

5. Now set your oven to 400°F.

6. Toss the cauliflower, remaining oil, and oregano together in a medium bowl. Arrange the cauliflower and chicken across a baking sheet in one layer.

7. Allow this to bake for 40 minutes. Stir the cauliflower and flip the chicken once during the cooking time. The chicken should be browned, and the juices should run clear. The temperature of the chicken should reach 165°F.

8. Serve with some lime juice. Enjoy!

Nutrition

- Calories: 175
- Protein: 16 g.
- Sodium: 77 mg.

- Potassium: 486 mg.
- Phosphorus: 152 mg.

7.17 RED AND GREEN GRAPES CHICKEN SALAD WITH CURRY

Preparation time: 5 minutes -Cooking time: 0 minute - Servings: 2

Ingredients

- 1 apple
- ¼ bowl of seedless, red grapes
- ¼ bowl of seedless, green grapes
- 4 cooked skinless and boneless chicken breasts
- 1 piece of celery

- ½ bowl of onion
- ½ bowl of canned water chestnuts
- ½ tsp. curry powder
- ¾ c. mayonnaise
- ⅛ tsp. black pepper

Directions

1. Cut the chicken into small dices and chop celery, onion, and apple. Drain and cut chestnuts.

2. Put together the chicken pieces, celery, onion, apple, grapes, water chestnuts, pepper, curry powder, and mayonnaise.

3. Serve it in a big salad bowl. Enjoy!

Nutrition

- Calories: 235
- Protein: 13 g.
- Sodium: 160 mg.

- Potassium: 200 mg.
- Phosphorus: 115 mg.

7.18 GRILLED CHICKEN PIZZA

Preparation time: 20 minutes - Cooking time: 15 minutes - Servings: 2

Ingredients

- 2 pita bread
- 3 tbsp. low-sodium BBQ sauce
- ¼ bowl of red onion

- 4 oz. cooked chicken
- 2 tbsp. crumbled Feta cheese
- ⅛ tsp. garlic powder

Directions

1. Preheat oven at 350°F (that is 175°C).
2. Place 2 pitas on the pan after you have put nonstick cooking spray on it.
3. Spread BBQ sauce (2 tbsps.) on the pita.
4. Cut the onion and put it on pita. Cube chicken and put it on the pitas.
5. Put also both Feta and the garlic powder over the pita.
6. Bake for 12 minutes. Serve and enjoy!

Nutrition

- Calories: 320
- Protein: 22 g.
- Sodium: 520 mg.
- Potassium: 250 mg.
- Phosphorus: 220 mg.

7.19 CHICKEN BREAST AND BOK CHOY

Preparation time: 10 minutes - Cooking time: 30 minutes - Servings: 4

Ingredients

- 4 slices of lemon
- Pepper, to taste
- 4 chicken breasts, boneless and skinless
- 1 tbsp. Dijon mustard
- 1 small leek, thinly sliced
- 2 julienned carrots
- 2 c. thinly sliced bok choy
- 1 tbsp. chopped thyme
- 1 tbsp. extra-virgin olive oil

Directions

1. Start by setting your oven to 425°F.
2. Mix the thyme, olive oil, and mustard in a small bowl.
3. Take 4 18-inch-long pieces of parchment paper and fold them in half. Cut them like you would make a heart. Open each of the pieces and lay them flat.
4. In each parchment piece, place ½ c. of bok choy, a few slices of leek, and a small handful of carrots.
5. Lay the chicken breast on top and season with some pepper.
6. Brush the chicken breasts with the marinade and top each one with a slice of lemon.
7. Fold the packets up, and roll down the edges to seal the packages.
8. Allow them to cook for 20 minutes. Let them rest for 5 minutes, and make sure you open them carefully when serving. Enjoy!

Nutrition

- Calories: 164
- Protein: 24 g.
- Phosphorus: 26 mg.
- Sodium: 356 mg.
- Potassium: 189 mg.

THE RENAL DIET COOKBOOK

7.20   BAKED HERBED CHICKEN

Preparation time: 10 minutes - Cooking time: 60 minutes - Servings: 6

Ingredients

- ¼ tsp. pepper
- 6 chicken thighs, bone-in
- 1 tbsp. chopped oregano
- 1 tsp. lemon zest
- 1 tbsp. chopped parsley
- 4 garlic cloves, minced
- 4 tbsp. butter at room temperature

Directions

1. Start by setting your oven to 425°F.
2. Add the lemon zest, parsley, oregano, garlic, and butter to a small bowl and mix well, making sure that everything is distributed evenly throughout the butter.
3. Lay the chicken on a baking pan and gently pull the skin back, but leaving it attached.
4. Brush the thigh meat with butter mixture and lay the skin back over the meat. Sprinkle on some pepper.
5. Bake the chicken for 40 minutes. The skin should be crispy, and the juices should be clear. Also, the chicken should reach 165°F.
6. Allow the chicken to rest for 5 minutes before serving. Enjoy!

Nutrition

- Calories: 226
- Protein: 16 g.
- Sodium: 120 mg.
- Potassium: 158 mg.
- Phosphorus: 114 mg.

CHAPTER 8 - SALAD RECIPES

8.1   PEAR AND BRIE SALAD

Preparation time: 5 minutes - Cooking time: 0 minutes - Servings: 4

Ingredients

- 1 tbsp. olive oil
- 1 c. arugula
- ½ lemon juice
- ½ c. canned pears
- ¼ cucumber
- ¼ c. chopped brie
- ½ tbsp. Black pepper to taste

Directions

1. Peel and dice the cucumber.
2. Dice the pear.
3. Wash the arugula.
4. Combine salad in a serving bowl and crumble the brie over the top.
5. Whisk the olive oil and lemon juice together.
6. Drizzle over the salad.
7. Season with a little black pepper to taste and serve immediately.

Nutrition

- Calories: 54
- Protein: 1 g.
- Carbohydrates: 12 g.
- Fat: 7 g.
- Sodium: 57 mg.
- Potassium: 115 mg.
- Phosphorus: 67 mg.

8.2   CAESAR SALAD

Preparation time: 5 minutes - Cooking time: 5 minutes - Servings: 4

Ingredients

- 1 head romaine lettuce
- ¼ c. mayonnaise
- 1 tbsp. lemon juice
- 4 anchovy fillets
- 1 tsp. Worcestershire sauce
- Black pepper to taste
- 5 garlic cloves
- 4 tbsps. Parmesan cheese
- 1 tsp. mustard

Directions

- In a bowl mix all ingredients and mix well.
- Serve with dressing.

Nutrition

- Calories: 44
- Fat: 2.1 g.
- Sodium: 83 mg.
- Potassium: 216 mg.
- Carbohydrates: 4.3 g.
- Protein: 3.2 g.
- Phosphorus: 45.6 mg.

8.3   THAI CUCUMBER SALAD

Preparation time: 5 minutes - Cooking time: 5 minutes - Servings: 2

Ingredients

- ¼ c. chopped peanuts
- ¼ c. white sugar
- ½ c. cilantro
- ¼ c. rice wine vinegar
- 3 cucumbers
- 2 jalapeño peppers

Directions

1. In a bowl add all ingredients and mix well.
2. Serve with dressing.

Nutrition

- Calories: 20
- Fat: 0 g.
- Sodium: 85 mg.
- Phosphorus: 46.8 mg.
- Carbohydrates: 5 g.
- Protein: 1 g.
- Potassium: 190.4 mg.

8.4 BROCCOLI-CAULIFLOWER SALAD

Preparation time: 5 minutes - Cooking time: 5 minutes - Servings: 4

Ingredients

- 1 tbsp. wine vinegar
- 1 c. cauliflower florets
- ¼ c. white sugar
- 2 c. hard-cooked eggs
- 5 slices bacon
- 1 c. broccoli florets
- 1 c. Cheddar cheese
- 1 c. mayonnaise

Directions

1. In a bowl add all ingredients and mix well.
2. Serve with dressing.

Nutrition

- Calories: 89.8
- Fat: 4.5 g.
- Sodium: 51.2 mg.
- Potassium: 257.6 mg.
- Carbohydrates: 11.5 g.
- Protein: 3.0 g.
- Phosphorus: 47 mg.

8.5 GREEN BEAN AND POTATO SALAD

Preparation time: 5 minutes - Cooking time: 5 minutes - Servings: 4

Ingredients

- ½ c. basil
- ¼ c. olive oil
- 1 tbsp. mustard
- ¾ lb. green beans
- 1 tbsp. lemon juice
- ½ c. balsamic vinegar
- 1 red onion
- 1 lb. red potatoes
- 1 garlic clove

Directions

1. Place potatoes in a pot with water and bring to a boil for 15–18 minutes or until tender.
2. Thrown in green beans after 5–6 minutes.
3. Drain and cut into cubes.
4. In a bowl add all ingredients and mix well.
5. Serve with dressing.

Nutrition

- Calories: 153.2
- Fat: 2.0 g.
- Sodium: 77.6 mg.
- Phosphorus: 49 mg.
- Potassium: 759.0 mg.
- Carbohydrates: 29.0 g.
- Protein: 6.9 g.

THE RENAL DIET COOKBOOK

8.6   ITALIAN CUCUMBER SALAD

Preparation time: 5 minutes - Cooking time: 0 minutes - Servings: 2

Ingredients

- ¼ c. rice vinegar
- ⅛ tsp. Stevia
- ½ tsp. olive oil
- ⅛ tsp. black pepper
- ½ cucumber, sliced
- 1 c. carrots, sliced
- 2 tbsps. green onion, sliced
- 2 tbsps. red bell pepper, sliced
- ½ tsp. Italian seasoning blend

Directions

1. Put all the salad ingredients into a suitable salad bowl.
2. Toss them well and refrigerate for 1 hour.
3. Serve.

Nutrition

- Calories: 112
- Total fat: 1.6 g.
- Cholesterol: 0 mg.
- Sodium: 43 mg.
- Protein: 2.3 g.
- Phosphorus: 198 mg.
- Potassium: 529 mg.

8.7   GRAPES JICAMA SALAD

Preparation time: 5 minutes - Cooking time: 0 minutes - Servings: 2

Ingredients

- 1 jicama, peeled and sliced
- 1 carrot, sliced
- ½ medium red onion, sliced
- 1 ¼ c. seedless grapes
- ⅓ c. fresh basil leaves
- 1 tbsp. apple cider vinegar
- 1 ½ tbsp. lemon juice
- 1 ½ tbsp. lime juice

Directions

1. Put all the salad ingredients into a suitable salad bowl.
2. Toss them well and refrigerate for 1 hour.
3. Serve.

Nutrition

- Calories: 203
- Total fat: 0.7 g.
- Sodium: 44 mg.
- Potassium: 429 mg.
- Protein: 3.7 g.
- Calcium: 79 mg.
- Phosphorus: 141 mg.

8.8   CUCUMBER COUSCOUS SALAD

Preparation time: 5 minutes - Cooking time: 0 minutes - Servings: 4

Ingredients

- 1 cucumber, sliced
- ½ c. red bell pepper, sliced
- ¼ c. sweet onion, sliced
- 2 tbsps. black olives, sliced
- ¼ c. parsley, chopped
- ½ c. couscous, cooked
- 2 tbsps. olive oil
- 2 tbsps. rice vinegar
- 2 tbsps. Feta cheese crumbled
- 1 ½ tsp. dried basil
- ¼ tsp. black pepper

Directions

1. Put all the salad ingredients into a suitable salad bowl.
2. Toss them well and refrigerate for 1 hour.
3. Serve.

Nutrition

- Calories: 202
- Total fat: 9.8 g.
- Sodium: 258 mg.
- Protein: 6.2 g.
- Calcium: 80 mg.
- Phosphorus: 192 mg.
- Potassium: 209 mg.

8.9   CARROT JICAMA SALAD

Preparation time: 5 minutes - Cooking time: 0 minutes - Servings: 2

Ingredients

- 2 c. carrots, julienned
- 1 ½ c. jicama, julienned
- 2 tbsps. lime juice
- 1 tbsp. olive oil
- ½ tbsp. apple cider
- ½ tsp. brown Swerve

Directions

1. Put all the salad ingredients into a suitable salad bowl.
2. Toss them well and refrigerate for 1 hour.
3. Serve.

Nutrition

- Calories: 173
- Total fat: 7.1 g.
- Sodium: 80 mg.
- Potassium: 501 mg.
- Protein: 1.6 g.
- Calcium: 50 mg.
- Phosphorus: 96 mg.

8.10 BUTTERSCOTCH APPLE SALAD

Preparation time: 5 minutes - Cooking time: 0 minutes - Servings: 6

Ingredients

- 3 c. jazz apples, chopped
- 8 oz. canned crushed pineapple
- 8 oz. whipped topping
- ½ c. butterscotch topping
- ⅓ c. almonds
- ¼ c. butterscotch chips

1. Directions
2. Put all the salad ingredients into a suitable salad bowl.
3. Toss them well and refrigerate for 1 hour.
4. Serve.

Nutrition

- Calories: 293
- Total fat: 12.7 g.
- Sodium: 52 mg.
- Protein: 4.2 g.
- Calcium: 65 mg.
- Phosphorus: 202 mg.
- Potassium: 296 mg.

8.11 CRANBERRY CABBAGE SLAW

Preparation time: 5 minutes - Cooking time: 0 minutes - Servings: 4

- Ingredients
- ½ medium cabbage head, shredded
- 1 medium red apple, shredded
- 2 tbsps. onion, sliced
- ½ c. dried cranberries
- ¼ c. almonds, toasted sliced
- ½ c. olive oil
- ¼ tsp. Stevia
- ¼ c. cider vinegar
- ½ tbsp. celery seed
- ½ tsp. dry mustard
- ½ c. cream

Directions

1. Take a suitable salad bowl.
2. Start tossing in all the ingredients.
3. Mix well and serve.

Nutrition

- Calories: 308
- Total fat: 24.5 g.
- Sodium: 23 mg.
- Potassium: 219 mg.
- Protein: 2.6 g.
- Calcium: 69 mg.
- Phosphorus: 257 mg.

THE RENAL DIET COOKBOOK

8.12 CHESTNUT NOODLE SALAD

Preparation time: 5 minutes - Cooking time: 0 minutes - Servings: 6

Ingredients

- 8 c. cabbage, shredded
- ½ c. canned chestnuts, sliced
- 6 green onions, chopped
- ¼ c. olive oil
- ¼ c. apple cider vinegar
- ¾ tsp. Stevia
- ⅛ tsp. black pepper
- 1 c. Chow Mein noodles, cooked

Directions

1. Take a suitable salad bowl.
2. Start tossing in all the ingredients.
3. Mix well and serve.

Nutrition

- Calories: 191
- Total fat: 13 g.
- Cholesterol: 1 mg.
- Sodium: 78 mg.
- Protein: 4.2 g.
- Calcium: 142 mg.
- Phosphorus: 188 mg.
- Potassium: 302 mg.

8.13 CRANBERRY BROCCOLI SALAD

Preparation time: 10 minutes - Cooking time: 0 minutes - Servings: 4

Ingredients

- ¾ c. plain Greek yogurt
- ¼ c. mayonnaise
- 2 tbsps. maple syrup
- 2 tbsps. apple cider vinegar
- 4 c. broccoli florets
- 1 medium apple, chopped
- ½ c. red onion, sliced
- ¼ c. parsley, chopped
- ½ c. dried cranberries
- ¼ c. pecans

Directions

1. Put all the salad ingredients into a suitable salad bowl.
2. Toss them well and refrigerate for 1 hour.
3. Serve.

Nutrition

- Calories: 252
- Total fat: 10.5 g.
- Saturated fat: 1.4 g.
- Cholesterol: 8 mg.
- Sodium: 157 mg.
- Protein: 9.4 g.
- Calcium: 106 mg.
- Phosphorus: 291 mg.
- Potassium: 480 mg.

THE RENAL DIET COOKBOOK

8.14 BALSAMIC BEET SALAD

Preparation time: 10 minutes - Cooking time: 0 minutes - Servings: 2

Ingredients

- 1 cucumber, peeled and sliced
- 15 oz. canned low-sodium beets, sliced
- 4 tsp. balsamic vinegar
- 2 tsp. sesame oil
- 2 tbsps. Gorgonzola cheese

Directions

1. Take a suitable salad bowl.
2. Start tossing in all the ingredients.
3. Mix well and serve.

Nutrition

- Calories: 145
- Total fat: 7.8 g.
- Saturated fat: 2.4 g.
- Cholesterol: 10 mg.
- Sodium: 426 mg.
- Protein: 5 g.
- Calcium: 109 mg.
- Phosphorus: 79 mg.
- Potassium: 229 mg.

8.15 SHRIMP SALAD

Preparation time: 8 minutes - Cooking time: 0 minutes - Servings: 4

Ingredients

- 1 lb. shrimp, boiled and chopped
- 1 hardboiled egg, chopped
- 1 tbsp. celery, chopped
- 1 tbsp. green pepper, chopped
- 1 tbsp. onion, chopped
- 2 tbsps. mayonnaise
- 1 tsp. lemon juice
- ½ tsp. chili powder
- ⅛ tsp. hot sauce
- ½ tsp. dry mustard
- Lettuce, chopped or shredded

Directions

1. Take a suitable salad bowl.
2. Start tossing in all the ingredients.
3. Mix well and serve.

Nutrition

- Calories: 184
- Total fat: 5.7 g.
- Saturated fat: 1.3 g.
- Cholesterol: 282 mg.
- Sodium: 381 mg.
- Protein: 27.5 g.
- Calcium: 114 mg.
- Phosphorus: 249 mg.
- Potassium: 233 mg.

8.16 CHICKEN CRANBERRY SAUCE SALAD

Preparation time: 10 minutes - Cooking time: 0 minutes - Servings: 6

Ingredients

- 3 c. chicken meat, cooked, cubed
- 1 c. grapes
- 2 c. carrots, shredded
- ¼ red onion, chopped
- 1 large yellow bell pepper, chopped
- ¼ c. mayonnaise
- ½ c. cranberry sauce

Directions

1. Put all the salad ingredients into a suitable salad bowl.
2. Toss them well and refrigerate for 1 hour.
3. Serve.

Nutrition

- Calories: 240
- Total fat: 8.6 g.
- Saturated fat: 1.9 g.
- Cholesterol: 65 mg.
- Sodium: 161 mg.
- Protein: 21 g.
- Calcium: 31 mg.
- Phosphorus: 260 mg.
- Potassium: 351 mg.

8.17 EGG CELERY SALAD

Preparation time: 10 minutes - Cooking time: 0 minutes - Servings: 4

Ingredients

- 4 eggs, boiled, peeled, and chopped
- ¼ c. celery, chopped
- ½ c. sweet onion, chopped
- 2 tbsps. sweet pickle, chopped
- 3 tbsps. mayonnaise
- 1 tbsp. mustard

Directions

Put all the salad ingredients into a suitable salad bowl.

Toss them well and refrigerate for 1 hour.

Serve.

Nutrition

- Calories: 134
- Total fat: 8.9 g.
- Saturated fat: 2.1 g.
- Cholesterol: 189 mg.
- Sodium: 259 mg.
- Protein: 6.8 g.
- Calcium: 36 mg.
- Phosphorus: 357 mg.
- Potassium: 113 mg.

8.18 CHICKEN ORANGE SALAD

Preparation time: 10 minutes - Cooking time: 0 minutes - Servings: 4

Ingredients

- 1 ½ c. chicken, cooked and diced
- ½ c. celery, diced
- ½ c. green pepper, chopped
- ¼ c. onion, sliced
- 1 c. orange, peeled and cut into segments
- ¼ c. mayonnaise
- ½ tsp. black pepper

Directions

1. Take a suitable salad bowl.
2. Start tossing in all the ingredients.
3. Mix well and serve.

Nutrition

- Calories: 167
- Total fat: 6.6 g.
- Saturated fat: 1.2 g.
- Cholesterol: 44 mg.
- Sodium: 151 mg.
- Protein: 16 g.
- Calcium: 25 mg.
- Phosphorus: 211 mg.
- Potassium: 249 mg.

8.19 ALMOND PASTA SALAD

Preparation time: 10 minutes - Cooking time: 0 minutes - Servings: 14

Ingredients

- 1 lb. elbow macaroni, cooked
- ½ c. sun-dried tomatoes, diced
- 1 (15 oz.) can whole artichokes, diced
- 1 orange bell pepper, diced
- 3 green onions, sliced
- 2 tbsps. basil, sliced
- 2 oz. slivered almonds

For the dressing:

- 1 garlic clove, minced
- 1 tbsp. Dijon mustard
- 1 tbsp. raw honey
- ¼ c. white balsamic vinegar
- ⅓ c. olive oil

Directions

1. Take a suitable salad bowl.
2. Start tossing in all the ingredients.
3. Mix well and serve.

Nutrition

- Calories: 260
- Total fat: 7.7 g.
- Saturated fat: 0.8 g.
- Cholesterol: 0 mg.
- Sodium: 143 mg.

- Protein: 9.6 g.
- Calcium: 44 mg.
- Phosphorus: 39 mg.
- Potassium: 585 mg.

8.20   PINEAPPLE BERRY SALAD

Preparation time: 10 minutes - Cooking time: 0 minutes - Servings: 4

Ingredients

- 4 c. pineapple, peeled and cubed
- 3 c. strawberries, chopped
- ¼ c. honey

- ½ c. basil leaves
- 1 tbsp. lemon zest
- ½ c. blueberries

Directions

1. Take a suitable salad bowl.
2. Start tossing in all the ingredients.
3. Mix well and serve.

Nutrition

- Calories: 128
- Total fat: 0.6 g.
- Saturated fat: 0 g.
- Cholesterol: 0 mg.
- Sodium: 3 mg.

- Protein: 1.8 g.
- Calcium: 40 mg.
- Phosphorus: 151 mg.
- Potassium: 362 mg.

CHAPTER 9 - DESSERT RECIPES

9.1   CHOCOLATE TRIFLE

Preparation time: 20 minutes - Cooking time: 15 minutes - Servings: 4

Ingredients

- 1 small plain sponge Swiss roll
- 3 oz. custard powder
- 5 oz. hot water
- 16 oz. canned mandarins
- 3 tbsps. cherry
- 5 oz. double cream
- 4 chocolate squares, grated

Directions

1. Whisk the custard powder with water in a bowl until dissolved.
2. In a bowl, mix the custard well until it becomes creamy and let it sit for 15 minutes.
3. Spread the Swiss roll and cut it into 4 squares.
4. Place the Swiss roll in the 4 serving cups.
5. Top the Swiss roll with mandarin, custard, cream, chocolate, and cherry.
6. Serve.

Nutrition

- Calories: 315
- Total fat: 13.5 g.
- Cholesterol: 43 mg.
- Sodium: 185 mg.
- Protein: 2.9 g.
- Calcium: 61 mg.
- Phosphorus: 184 mg.
- Potassium: 129 mg.

9.2   PINEAPPLE MERINGUES

Preparation time: 10 minutes - Cooking time: 0 minutes - Servings: 4

Ingredients

- 4 meringue nests
- 8 oz. Crème Fraiche
- 2 oz. stem ginger, chopped
- 8 oz. can pineapple chunks

Directions

1. Place the meringue nests on the serving plates.
2. Whisk the ginger with Crème Fraiche and pineapple chunks.
3. Divide the pineapple mixture over the meringue nests.
4. Serve.

Nutrition

- Calories: 312
- Cholesterol: 0 mg.
- Sodium: 41 mg.
- Protein: 2.3 g.
- Calcium: 3 mg.
- Phosphorus: 104 mg.
- Potassium: 110 mg.

9.3   BAKED CUSTARD

Preparation time: 15 minutes - Cooking time: 30 minutes -Servings: 1

Ingredients

- ½ c. milk
- 1 egg, beaten
- ⅛ tsp. nutmeg
- ⅛ tsp. vanilla
- Sweetener to taste
- ½ c. water

Directions

1. Lightly warm up the milk in a pan, then whisk in the egg, nutmeg, vanilla, and sweetener.
2. Pour this custard mixture into a ramekin.
3. Place the ramekin in a baking pan and pour ½ c. water into the pan.
4. Bake the custard for 30 minutes at 325°F.
5. Serve fresh.

Nutrition

- Calories: 127
- Total fat: 7 g.
- Cholesterol: 174 mg.
- Potassium: 171 mg.
- Sodium: 119 mg.
- Calcium: 169 mg.
- Phosphorus: 309 mg.

9.4   APPLE CRISP

Preparation time: 20 minutes - Cooking time: 45 minutes - Servings: 6

Ingredients

- 4 c. apples, peeled and chopped
- ½ tsp. Stevia
- 3 tbsps. brandy
- 2 tsps. lemon juice
- ½ tsp. cinnamon
- ⅛ tsp. nutmeg
- ¾ c. dry oats
- ¼ c. brown Swerve
- 2 tbsps. flour
- 2 tbsps. butter

Directions

1. Toss the oats with the flour, butter, and brown Swerve in a bowl and keep it aside.
2. Whisk the remaining crisp ingredients in an 8-inch baking pan.
3. Spread the oats mixture over the crispy filling.
4. Bake it for 45 minutes at 350°F in a preheated oven.
5. Slice and serve.

Nutrition

- Calories: 214
- Total fat: 4.8 g.
- Cholesterol: 0 mg.
- Sodium: 48 mg.
- Protein: 2.1 g.
- Calcium: 15 mg.
- Phosphorus: 348 mg.
- Potassium: 212 mg.

9.5   ALMOND COOKIES

Preparation time: 10 minutes - Cooking time: 12 minutes - Servings: 24

Ingredients

- 1 c. butter, softened
- 1 c. granulate Swerve
- 1 egg
- 3 c. flour
- 1 tsp. baking soda
- 1 tsp. almond extract

Directions

1. Beat the butter with the Swerve in a mixer then gradually stir in the remaining ingredients.
2. Mix well until it forms a cookie dough then divide the dough into small balls.
3. Spread each ball into ¾-inch rounds and place them on a cookie sheet.
4. Poke 2–3 holes in each cookie then bake for 12 minutes at 400°F.
5. Serve.

Nutrition

- Calories: 159
- Total fat: 7.9 g.
- Cholesterol: 7 mg.
- Sodium: 144 mg.
- Protein: 1.9 g.
- Calcium: 6 mg.
- Phosphorus: 274 mg.
- Potassium: 23 mg.

9.6   LIME PIE

Preparation time: 10 minutes - Cooking time: 5 minutes - Servings: 8

Ingredients

- 5 tbsps. butter, unsalted
- 1 ¼ c. cracker crumbs
- ¼ c. granulated Swerve
- ⅓ c. lime juice
- 14 oz. condensed milk
- 1 c. heavy whipping cream
- 1 (9-inch) pie shell

Directions

1. Switch on your gas oven and preheat it to 350°F.
2. Whisk the cracker crumbs with the Swerve and melted butter in a suitable bowl.
3. Spread this cracker crumbs crust in a 9-inch pie shell and bake it for 5 minutes.
4. Meanwhile, mix the condensed milk with the lime juice in a bowl.
5. Whisk the heavy cream in a mixer until foamy, then add in the condensed milk mixture.
6. Mix well, then spread this filling in the baked crust.
7. Refrigerate the pie for 4 hours.
8. Slice and serve.

Nutrition

- Calories: 391
- Total fat: 22.4 g.
- Cholesterol: 57 mg.
- Sodium: 52 mg.
- Protein: 5.3 g.
- Calcium: 163 mg.
- Phosphorus: 199 mg.
- Potassium: 221 mg.

9.7   BUTTERY LEMON SQUARES

Preparation time: 10 minutes - Cooking time: 35 minutes - Servings: 12

Ingredients

- 1 c. refined Swerve
- 1 c. flour
- ½ c. butter, unsalted
- 1 c. granulated Swerve
- ½ tsp. baking powder
- 2 eggs, beaten
- 4 tbsps. lemon juice
- 1 tbsp. butter, unsalted, softened
- 1 tbsp. lemon zest

Directions

1. Start mixing ¼ c. refined Swerve, ½ c. butter, and flour in a bowl.
2. Spread this crust mixture in an 8-inch square pan and press it.
3. Bake this flour crust for 15 minutes at 350°F.
4. Meanwhile, prepare the filling by beating 2 tbsps. lemon juice, ¼ c. granulated Swerve, eggs, lemon zest, and baking powder in a mixer.

5. Spread this filling in the baked crust and bake again for about 20 minutes.

6. Meanwhile, prepare the squares' icing by beating 2 tbsps. lemon juice, 1 tbsp. butter, and ¾ c. refine Swerve.

7. Once the lemon pie is baked well, allow it to cool.

8. Sprinkle the icing mixture on top of the lemon pie then cut it into 36 squares.

9. Serve.

Nutrition

- Calories: 229
- Total fat: 9.5 g.
- Cholesterol: 50 mg.
- Sodium: 66 mg.

- Protein: 2.1 g.
- Calcium: 18 mg.
- Phosphorus: 257 mg.
- Potassium: 51 mg.

9.8   BLACKBERRY CREAM CHEESE PIE

Preparation time: 15 minutes - Cooking time: 45 minutes - Servings: 8

Ingredients

- ⅓ c. butter, unsalted
- 4 c. blackberries
- 1 tsp. Stevia

- 1 c. flour
- ½ tsp. baking powder
- ¾ c. cream cheese

Directions

1. Switch your gas oven to 375°F to preheat.
2. Layer a 2-quart baking dish with melted butter.
3. Mix the blackberries with Stevia in a small bowl.
4. Beat the remaining ingredients in a mixer until they form a smooth batter.
5. Evenly spread this pie batter in the prepared baking dish and top it with blackberries.
6. Bake the blackberry pie for about 45 minutes in the preheated oven.
7. Slice and serve once chilled.

Nutrition

- Calories: 239
- Total fat: 8.4 g.
- Cholesterol: 20 mg.
- Sodium: 63 mg.
- Potassium: 170 mg.

- Protein: 2.8 g.
- Calcium: 67 mg.
- Phosphorus: 105 mg.

9.9   APPLE CINNAMON PIE

Preparation time: 20 minutes - Cooking time: 50 minutes - Servings: 12

Ingredients

For the apple filling:

- 9 c. apples, peeled, cored, and sliced
- 1 tbsp. Stevia
- ⅓ c. all-purpose flour
- 2 tbsps. lemon juice
- 1 tsp. ground cinnamon
- 2 tbsps. butter

For the pie dough:

- 2 ¼ c. all-purpose flour
- 1 tsp. Stevia
- 1 ½ sticks unsalted butter
- 6 oz. cream cheese
- 3 tbsps. cold heavy whipping cream
- Water, if needed

Directions

1. Start by preheating your gas oven at 425°F.
2. For the apple filling: Mix the apple slices with cinnamon, 1 tbsp. of butter, lemon juice, flour, and Stevia in a bowl and keep it aside covered.
3. For the pie dough: Whisk the flour with Stevia, butter, cream cheese, and cream in a mixing bowl to form the dough.
4. If the dough is too dry, slowly add some water to make a smooth dough ball.
5. Cut the dough into 2 equal-size pieces and spread them into a 9-inch sheet.
6. Place one of the sheets at the bottom of a 9-inch pie pan.
7. Evenly spread the apples in this pie shell and add 1 tbsp. of butter over it.
8. Cover the apple filling with the second sheet of the dough and pinch down the edges.
9. Make 1-inch-deep cuts on top of the pie and bake for about 50 minutes until golden.
10. Slice and serve.

Nutrition

- Calories: 303
- Total fat: 8.8 g.
- Cholesterol: 26 mg.
- Sodium: 30 mg.
- Protein: 4.2 g.
- Calcium: 21 mg.
- Phosphorus: 381 mg.
- Potassium: 229 mg.

9.10   MAPLE CRISP BARS

Preparation time: 10 minutes - Cooking time: 5 minutes - Servings: 20

Ingredients

- ⅓ c. butter
- 1 c. brown Swerve
- 1 tsp. maple extract
- ½ c. maple syrup
- 8 c. puffed rice cereal

Directions

1. Mix the butter with Swerve, maple extract, and syrup in a saucepan over moderate heat.
2. Cook by slowly stirring this mixture for 5 minutes then toss in the rice cereal.
3. Mix well, then press this cereal mixture in a 13x9-inch baking dish.
4. Refrigerate the mixture for 2 hours then cut into 20 bars.
5. Serve.

Nutrition

- Calories: 107
- Total fat: 3.1 g.
- Cholesterol: 0 mg.
- Sodium: 36 mg.

- Protein: 0.4 g.
- Calcium: 7 mg.
- Phosphorus: 233 mg.
- Potassium: 24 mg.

9.11   PINEAPPLE GELATIN PIE

Preparation time: 10 minutes - Cooking time: 5 minutes - Servings: 8

Ingredients

- ⅔ c. graham cracker crumbs
- 2 ½ tbsps. butter, melted
- 1 (20 oz.) can crushed pineapple, juice packed

- 1 small gelatin pack
- 1 tbsp. lemon juice
- 2 egg whites, pasteurized
- ¼ tsp. cream of tartar

Directions

1. Whisk the crumbs with the butter in a bowl then spread them onto an 8-inch pie plate.
2. Bake the crust for 5 minutes at 425°F.
3. Meanwhile, mix the pineapple juice with the gelatin in a saucepan.
4. Place it over low heat then add the pineapple and lemon juice. Mix well.
5. Beat the cream of tartar and egg whites in a mixer until creamy.
6. Add the cooked pineapple mixture then mix well.
7. Spread this filling in the baked crust.
8. Refrigerate the pie for 4 hours then slice.
9. Serve.

Nutrition

- Calories: 106
- Total fat: 4.2 g.
- Cholesterol: 0 mg.
- Sodium: 117 mg.
- Potassium: 33 mg.

- Protein: 2.2 g.
- Calcium: 3 mg.
- Phosphorus: 231 mg.

9.12 CHOCOLATE GELATIN MOUSSE

Preparation time: 10 minutes - Cooking time: 5 minutes - Servings: 4

- Ingredients
- 1 tsp. Stevia
- ½ tsp. gelatin
- ¼ c. milk
- ½ c. chocolate chips
- 1 tsp. vanilla
- ½ c. heavy cream, whipped

Directions

1. Whisk the Stevia with the gelatin and milk in a saucepan and cook up to a boil.
2. Stir in the chocolate and vanilla then mix well until it has completely melted.
3. Beat the cream in a mixer until fluffy then fold in the chocolate mixture.
4. Mix it gently with a spatula then transfer to the serving bowl.
5. Refrigerate the dessert for 4 hours.
6. Serve.

Nutrition

- Calories: 200
- Total fat: 12.1 g.
- Cholesterol: 27 mg.
- Sodium: 31 mg.
- Protein: 3.2 g.
- Calcium: 68 mg.
- Phosphorus: 120 mg.
- Potassium: 100 mg.

9.13 CHEESECAKE BITES

Preparation time: 10 minutes - Cooking time: 5 minutes - Servings: 16

Ingredients

- 8 oz. cream cheese
- ½ tsp. vanilla
- ¼ c. Swerve

Directions

1. Add all ingredients into the mixing bowl and blend until well combined.
2. Place bowl into the fridge for 1 hour.
3. Remove bowl from the fridge. Make small balls from the cheese mixture and place them on a baking dish.
4. Serve and enjoy.

Nutrition

- Calories: 50
- Fat: 4.9 g.
- Carbohydrates: 0.4 g.
- Cholesterol: 16 mg.
- Sugar: 0.1 g.
- Protein: 1.1 g.

9.14 PUMPKIN BITES

Preparation time: 10 minutes -Cooking time: 5 minutes - Servings: 12

Ingredients

- 8 oz. cream cheese
- 1 tsp. vanilla
- 1 tsp. pumpkin pie spice
- ¼ c. coconut flour
- ¼ c. Erythritol
- ½ c. pumpkin puree
- 4 oz. butter

Directions

1. Add all ingredients into the mixing bowl and beat using a hand mixer until well combined.
2. Scoop mixture into the silicone ice cube tray and place it in the refrigerator until set.
3. Serve and enjoy.

Nutrition

- Calories: 149
- Fat: 14.6 g.
- Carbohydrates: 8.1 g.
- Sugar: 5.4 g.
- Protein: 2 g.
- Cholesterol: 41 mg.

9.15 PROTEIN BALLS

Preparation time: 5 minutes - Cooking time: 5 minutes - Servings: 12

Ingredients

- ¾ c. peanut butter
- 1 tsp. cinnamon
- 3 tbsp. Erythritol
- 1 ½ c. almond flour

Directions

1. Add all ingredients into the mixing bowl and blend until well combined.
2. Place bowl into the fridge for 30 minutes.
3. Remove bowl from the fridge. Make small balls from the mixture and place them on a baking dish.
4. Serve and enjoy.

Nutrition

- Calories: 179
- Fat: 14.8 g.
- Carbohydrates: 10.1 g.
- Cholesterol: 0 mg.
- Sugar: 5.3 g.
- Protein: 7 g.

9.16 CASHEW CHEESE BITES

Preparation time: 5 minutes - Cooking time: 5 minutes - Servings: 12

Ingredients

- 8 oz. cream cheese
- 1 tsp. cinnamon
- 1 c. cashew butter

Directions

1. Add all ingredients into the blender and blend until smooth.
2. Pour blended mixture into the mini muffin liners and place them in the refrigerator until set.
3. Serve and enjoy.

Nutrition

- Calories: 192
- Fat: 17.1 g.
- Carbohydrates: 6.5 g.
- Sugar: 0 g.
- Protein: 5.2 g.
- Cholesterol: 21 mg.

9.17 HEALTHY CINNAMON LEMON TEA

Preparation time: 5 minutes - Cooking time: 5 minutes - Servings: 1

Ingredients

- ½ tbsp. fresh lemon juice
- 1 c. water
- 1 tsp. ground cinnamon

Directions

1. Add water in a saucepan and bring to boil over medium heat.
2. Add cinnamon and stir to cinnamon dissolve.
3. Add lemon juice and stir well.
4. Serve hot.

Nutrition

- Calories: 9
- Fat: 0.2 g.
- Carbohydrates: 2 g.
- Cholesterol: 0 mg.
- Sugar: 0.3 g.
- Protein: 0.2 g.

9.18 APPLE PIE

Preparation time: 10 minutes - Cooking time: 50 minutes - Servings: 6

Ingredients

- 6 medium apples, peeled, cored, and sliced
- ½ c. granulated sugar
- 1 tsp. ground cinnamon
- 1 tbsp. butter
- 2 ⅔ c. all-purpose flour
- 1 c. shortening
- 6 tbsp. water

Directions

1. Preheat your oven to 425°F.
2. Toss the apple slices with cinnamon and sugar in a bowl and set them aside covered.
3. Blend the flour with the shortening in a pastry blender then add chilled water by a spoon.
4. Continue mixing and adding the water until it forms a smooth dough ball.
5. Divide the dough into 2 equal-size pieces and spread them into 2 separate 9-inch sheets.
6. Arrange the sheet of dough at the bottom of a 9-inch pie pan.
7. Spread the apples in the pie shell and spread 1 tbsp. of butter over it.
8. Cover the filling with the remaining sheet of the dough and pinch down the edges.
9. Carve 1-inch cuts on top of the pie and bake for 50 minutes or more until golden.
10. Slice and serve.

Nutrition

- Calories: 517
- Protein: 4 g.
- Carbohydrates: 51 g.
- Fat: 33 g.
- Cholesterol: 24 mg.
- Sodium: 65 mg.
- Potassium: 145 mg.
- Phosphorus: 43 mg.
- Calcium: 24 mg.
- Fiber: 2.7 g.

9.19 BLUEBERRY CREAM CONES

Preparation time: 10 minutes - Cooking time: 0 minutes - Servings: 6

Ingredients

- 4 oz. cream cheese
- 1 ½ c. whipped topping
- 1 ¼ c. fresh or frozen blueberries
- ¼ c. blueberry jam or preserves
- 6 small ice cream cones

Directions

1. Start by softening the cream cheese then beat it in a mixer until fluffy.
2. Fold in jam and fruits.
3. Divide the mixture into the ice cream cones.
4. Serve fresh.

Nutrition

- Calories: 177
- Protein: 3 g.
- Carbohydrates: 21 g.
- Fat: 9 g.
- Cholesterol: 21 mg.
- Sodium: 95 mg.
- Potassium: 81 mg.
- Phosphorus: 40 mg.
- Calcium: 24 mg.
- Fiber: 1.0 g.

9.20   CHERRY COFFEE CAKE

Preparation time: 10 minutes - Cooking time: 40 minutes - Servings: 6

Ingredients

- ½ c. unsalted butter
- 2 eggs
- 1 c. granulated sugar
- 1 c. sour cream
- 1 tsp. vanilla
- 2 c. all-purpose white flour
- 1 tsp. baking powder
- 1 tsp. baking soda
- 20 oz. cherry pie filling

Directions

1. Preheat oven to 350°F.
2. Soften the butter first then beat it with the eggs, sugar, vanilla, and sour cream in a mixer.
3. Separately mix flour with baking soda and baking powder.
4. Add this mixture to the egg mixture and mix well until smooth.
5. Spread this batter evenly in a 9x13-inch baking pan.
6. Bake the pie for 40 minutes in the oven until golden on the surface.
7. Slice and serve with cherry pie filling on top.

Nutrition

- Calories: 204
- Protein: 3 g.
- Carbohydrates: 30 g.
- Fat: 8 g.
- Cholesterol: 43 mg.
- Sodium: 113 mg.
- Potassium: 72 mg.
- Phosphorus: 70 mg.
- Calcium: 41 mg.
- Fiber: 0.5 g.

CHAPTER 10 - SMOOTHIES AND DRINKS RECIPES

10.1   ALMONDS AND BLUEBERRIES SMOOTHIE

Preparation time: 5 minutes - Cooking time: 3 minutes - Servings: 2

Ingredients

- ¼ c. ground almonds, unsalted
- 1 c. fresh blueberries
- Fresh juice of a 1 lemon
- 1 c. fresh kale leaf
- ½ c. coconut water
- 1 c. water
- 2 tbsp. plain yogurt (optional)

Directions

1. Dump all ingredients in your high-speed blender, and blend until your smoothie is smooth.
2. Pour the mixture into a chilled glass.
3. Serve and enjoy!

Nutrition

- Calories: 110
- Carbohydrates: 8 g.
- Protein: 2 g.
- Fat: 7 g.
- Fiber: 2 g.
- Calcium: 19 mg.
- Phosphorus: 16 mg.
- Potassium: 27 mg.
- Sodium: 101 mg.

10.2 ALMONDS AND ZUCCHINI SMOOTHIE

Preparation time: 5 minutes - Cooking time: 3 minutes - Servings: 2

Ingredients

- 1 c. zucchini, cooked and mashed, unsalted
- 1 ½ c. almond milk
- 1 tbsp. almond butter, plain, unsalted
- 1 tsp. pure almond extract
- 2 tbsp. ground almonds or macadamia almonds
- ½ c. water
- 1 c. ice cubes crushed (optional, for serving)

Directions

1. Dump all ingredients from the list above in your fast-speed blender; blend for 45–60 seconds or to taste.
2. Serve with crushed ice.

Nutrition

- Calories: 322
- Carbohydrates: 6 g.
- Protein: 6 g.
- Fat: 30 g.
- Fiber: 3.5 g
- Calcium: 9 mg.
- Phosphorus: 26 mg.
- Potassium: 27 mg.
- Sodium: 121 mg.

10.3 BLUEBERRIES AND COCONUT SMOOTHIE

Preparation time: 5 minutes - Cooking time: 3 minutes - Servings: 5

Ingredients

- 1 c. frozen blueberries, unsweetened
- 1 c. Stevia or Erythritol sweetener
- 2 c. coconut milk (canned)
- 1 c. fresh spinach leaves
- 2 tbsp. shredded coconut (unsweetened)
- ¾ c. water

Directions

1. Place all ingredients from the list in the food processor or in your strong blender.
2. Blend for 45–60 seconds or to taste.
3. Ready to drink! Serve!

Nutrition

- Calories: 190
- Carbohydrates: 8 g.
- Protein: 3 g.
- Fat: 18 g.
- Fiber: 2 g.
- Calcium: 79 mg.
- Phosphorus: 216 mg.
- Potassium: 207 mg.
- Sodium: 121 mg.

10.4 CREAMY DANDELION GREENS AND CELERY SMOOTHIE

Preparation time: 10 minutes - Cooking time: 3 minutes - Servings: 2

Ingredients

- 1 handful of raw dandelion greens
- 2 celery sticks
- 2 tbsp. chia seeds
- 1 small piece of ginger, minced
- ½ c. almond milk
- ½ c. water
- ½ c. plain yogurt

Directions

1. Rinse and clean dandelion leaves from any dirt; add in a high-speed blender.
2. Clean the ginger; keep only the inner part and cut in small slices; add in a blender.
3. Blend all remaining ingredients until smooth.
4. Serve and enjoy!

Nutrition

- Calories: 58
- Carbohydrates: 5 g.
- Protein: 3 g.
- Fat: 6 g.
- Fiber: 3 g
- Calcium: 29 mg.
- Phosphorus: 76 mg.
- Potassium: 27 mg.
- Sodium: 121 mg.

10.5 DARK TURNIP GREENS SMOOTHIE

Preparation time: 10 minutes - Cooking time: 3 minutes - Servings: 2

Ingredients

- 1 c. raw turnip greens
- 1 ½ c. almond milk
- 1 tbsp. almond butter
- ½ c. water
- ½ tsp. cocoa powder, unsweetened
- 1 tbsp. dark chocolate chips
- ¼ tsp. cinnamon
- 1 pinch of salt
- ½ c. crushed ice

Directions

1. Rinse and clean turnip greens from any dirt.
2. Place the turnip greens in your blender along with all other ingredients.
3. Blend it for 45–60 seconds or until done; smooth and creamy.
4. Serve with or without crushed ice.

Nutrition

- Calories: 131
- Carbohydrates: 6 g.
- Protein: 4 g.
- Fat: 10 g.
- Fiber: 2.5 g.

10.6 FRESH CUCUMBER, KALE AND RASPBERRY SMOOTHIE

Preparation time: 10 minutes - Cooking time: 3 minutes - Servings: 3

Ingredients

- 1 ½ c. cucumber, peeled
- ½ c. raw kale leaves
- 1 ½ c. fresh raspberries
- 1 c. almond milk
- 1 c. water
- Ice cubes crushed (optional)
- 2 tbsp. natural sweetener (Stevia, Erythritol, etc.)

Directions

1. Place all ingredients listed in a high-speed blender; blend for 35–40 Seconds.
2. Serve into chilled glasses.
3. Add more natural sweeter if you like. Enjoy!

Nutrition

- Calories: 70
- Carbohydrates: 8 g.
- Protein: 3 g.
- Fat: 6 g.
- Fiber: 5 g.

10.7 GREEN COCONUT SMOOTHIE

Preparation time: 10 minutes - Cooking time: 3 minutes - Servings: 2

Ingredients

- 1 ¼ c. coconut milk (canned)
- 2 tbsp. chia seeds
- 1 c. fresh kale leaves
- 1 c. spinach leaves
- 1 scoop vanilla protein powder
- 1 c. ice cubes
- Granulated Stevia sweetener (to taste; optional)
- ½ c. water

Directions

1. Rinse and clean kale and the spinach leaves from any dirt.
2. Add all ingredients to your blender.
3. Blend until you get a nice smoothie.
4. Serve into chilled glass.

Nutrition

- Calories: 179
- Carbohydrates: 5 g.
- Protein: 4 g.
- Fat: 18 g.
- Fiber: 2.5 g.
- Calcium: 22 mg.
- Phosphorus: 46 mg.
- Potassium: 34 mg.
- Sodium: 131 mg.

10.8 RASPBERRY SMOOTHIE

Preparation time: 4 minutes - Cooking time: 0 minutes - Servings: 1

Ingredients

- 1 c. frozen raspberries
- 1 medium peach, pitted, sliced
- ½ c. tofu
- 1 tbsp. honey
- 1 c. milk

Directions

1. First, begin by putting everything into a blender jug.
2. Pulse it for 30 seconds until well blended.
3. Serve chilled.

Nutrition

- Calories: 223
- Total fat: 2.7 g.
- Saturated fat: 0.3 g.
- Cholesterol: 0 mg.
- Sodium: 99 mg.
- Carbohydrates: 49.9 g.
- Dietary fiber: 7.2 g.
- Sugar: 43.1 g.
- Protein: 3.6 g.
- Calcium: 176 mg.
- Phosphorus: 95 mg.
- Potassium: 426 mg.

10.9 SUNNY PINEAPPLE BREAKFAST SMOOTHIE

Preparation time: 5 minutes - Cooking time: 1 minute - Servings: 1

Ingredients

- ½ c. frozen pineapple chunks
- ⅔ c. almond milk
- ½ tsp. ginger powder
- 1 tbsp. agave syrup

Directions

1. Blend everything in a blender until nice and smooth (around 30 seconds).
2. Transfer into a tall glass or mason jar.
3. Serve and enjoy.

Nutrition

- Calories: 186
- Carbohydrates: 43.7 g.
- Protein: 2.28 g.
- Sodium: 130 mg.
- Fat: 2.3 g.
- Potassium: 135 mg.
- Phosphorus: 18 mg.
- Dietary fiber: 2.4 g.

10.10   BLUEBERRY BURST SMOOTHIE

Preparation time: 5 minutes - Cooking time: 0 minute - Servings: 2

Ingredients

- 1 c. blueberries
- 1 c. chopped collard greens
- 1 c. Homemade Rice Milk or unsweetened store-bought rice milk
- 1 tbsp. almond butter
- 3 ice cubes

Directions

1. In a blender, combine the blueberries, collard greens, milk, almond butter, and ice cubes.
2. Process until smooth, and serve.

Nutrition tip: Collard greens are a nutrient-dense food loaded with anticarcinogenic, antiviral, antibiotic, and antioxidant properties. Because collard greens are much lower in potassium than kale, they are a great substitute in recipes that call for its cruciferous cousin.

Nutrition

- Calories: 131
- Total fat: 6 g.
- Saturated fat: 0 g.
- Cholesterol: 0 mg.
- Carbohydrates: 19 g.
- Fiber: 3 g.
- Protein: 3 g.
- Phosphorus: 51 mg.
- Potassium: 146 mg.
- Sodium: 60 mg.

10.11   BLUEBERRY SMOOTHIE BOWL

Preparation time: 5 minutes - Cooking time: 0 minute - Servings: 1

Ingredients

- ½ c. frozen blueberries
- ½ c. vanilla-flavored almond milk
- 1 tbsp. agave syrup
- 1 tsp. chia seeds

Directions

1. Put all the ingredients in the blender except chia seeds, and blend until smooth. You should end up with a thick smoothie paste.
2. Transfer into a cereal bowl and top with chia seeds on top.

Nutrition

- Calories: 278.5
- Carbohydrates: 38.72 g.
- Protein: 1.3 g
- Sodium: 76.33 mg.
- Potassium: 229.1 mg.
- Phosphorus: 59.2 mg.
- Dietary fiber: 7.4 g.
- Fat: 6 g.

10.12   CUCUMBER SPINACH GREEN SMOOTHIE

Preparation time: 5 minutes - Cooking time: 0 minute - Servings: 2

Ingredients

- ½ cucumber, peeled and roughly chopped
- ½ green apple, roughly chopped
- 1 c. Homemade Rice Milk or unsweetened store-bought rice milk
- 2 c. spinach
- 3 ice cubes

Directions

1. In a blender, combine the cucumber, apple, milk, spinach, and ice.
2. Process until smooth, and serve.

Nutrition tip: A tart green apple is lovely in this smoothie, as it creates a subtle sweetness. However, if you prefer, other apples, such as Fuji, Red Delicious, or McIntosh, can be used. If you are using a thick-skinned apple, peel it first for a nicer texture in the finished smoothie.

Nutrition

- Calories: 75
- Total fat: 2 g.
- Saturated fat: 0 g.
- Cholesterol: 0 mg.
- Carbohydrates: 14 g.
- Fiber: 2 g.
- Protein: 1 g.
- Phosphorus: 34 mg.
- Potassium: 313 mg.
- Sodium: 81 mg.

10.13   WATERMELON KIWI SMOOTHIE

Preparation time: 5 minutes - Cooking time: 0 minute - Servings: 2

Ingredients

- 2 c. watermelon chunks
- 1 kiwifruit, peeled
- 1 c. ice

Directions

1. In a blender, combine the watermelon, kiwi, and ice.
2. Process until smooth.

Nutrition tip: While watermelon tastes particularly sweet, it has only half the sugar of an apple. Because sugar is the main taste-producing element, it stands out the most. The other primary ingredient in watermelon is water.

Nutrition

- Calories: 67
- Total fat: 0 g.
- Saturated fat: 0 g.
- Cholesterol: 0 mg.
- Carbohydrates: 17 g.
- Fiber: 2 g.
- Protein: 1 g.
- Phosphorus: 28 mg.
- Potassium: 278 mg.
- Sodium: 3 mg.

10.14   MINT LASSI

Preparation time: 5 minutes - Cooking time: 0 minute - Servings: 2

Ingredients

- 1 tsp. cumin seeds
- ½ c. mint leaves
- 1 c. plain, unsweetened yogurt
- ½ c. water

Directions

1. In a skillet, toast cumin seeds until fragrant, 1–2 minutes in medium heat.
2. Transfer the seeds to a blender, along with the mint, yogurt, and water, and process until smooth.

Nutrition tip: If you prefer the flavor of cilantro over mint, try it here instead. Another great substitute is to use ½ c. of strawberries along with ¼ tsp. of ground cardamom instead of the mint.

Nutrition

- Calories: 114
- Total fat: 6 g.
- Saturated fat: 3 g.
- Cholesterol: 15 mg.
- Carbohydrates: 5 g.
- Fiber: 0 g.
- Protein: 10 g.
- Phosphorus: 158 mg.
- Potassium: 179 mg.
- Sodium: 43 mg.

10.15   FENNEL DIGESTIVE COOLER

Preparation time: 5 minutes - Cooking time: 15 minutes - Servings: 2

Ingredients

- 2 c. Homemade Rice Milk or unsweetened store-bought rice milk
- ¼ c. fennel seeds, ground
- ¼ tsp. ground cloves
- 1 tbsp. honey

Directions

1. In a blender, combine the milk, fennel seeds, cloves, and honey.
2. Process until smooth, and let rest for 30 minutes.
3. Pour over a wire mesh strainer lined with cheesecloth or over a coffee filter set over a glass or jar.
4. Serve.

Nutrition tip: Fennel is a warming herb that is supportive of treating indigestion, gas, and hypertension. High in quercetin, an antioxidant flavonoid, fennel fights inflammation and inhibits the development of cancer, among other benefits.

Nutrition

- Calories: 163
- Total fat: 2 g.
- Saturated fat: 0 g.
- Cholesterol: 0 mg.
- Carbohydrates: 30 g.
- Fiber: 5 g.

- Protein: 3 g.
- Phosphorus: 57 mg.

- Potassium: 205 mg.
- Sodium: 141 mg.

10.16   CINNAMON HORCHATA

Preparation time: 5 minutes - Cooking time: 0 minute - Servings: 5

Ingredients

- 1 c. long-grain white rice
- 4 c. water
- 1 cinnamon stick, broken into pieces
- 1 c. Homemade Rice Milk or unsweetened store-bought rice milk

- 1 tsp. vanilla extract
- 1 tsp. ground cinnamon
- ⅓ c. granulated sugar

Directions

1. Using a blender, mix the rice, water, and cinnamon stick pieces. For about 1 minute, blend until the rice begins to break up. Let stand at room temperature for at least 3 hours or overnight.
2. Place a wire mesh strainer over a pitcher, and pour the liquid into it. Discard the rice.
3. Add the milk, vanilla, ground cinnamon, and sugar. Stir to combine.
4. Serve over ice.

Nutrition tip: For an even richer flavor, add 1 tbsp. of unsweetened cocoa powder to the horchata with the ground cinnamon in Step 3.

Nutrition

- Calories: 123
- Total fat: 2 g.
- Saturated fat: 0 g.
- Cholesterol: 0 mg.
- Carbohydrates: 26 g.
- Sodium: 32 mg.

- Fiber: 0 g.
- Protein: 1 g.
- Phosphorus: 34 mg.
- Potassium: 78 mg.

10.17   VANILLA CHIA SMOOTHIE

Preparation time: 5 minutes - Cooking time: 5 minutes - Servings: 2

Ingredients

- 1 c. Homemade Rice Milk or unsweetened store-bought rice milk
- 2 black tea bags
- 1 tsp. vanilla extract
- 1 c. ice
- 1 tsp. honey
- 2 tbsps. chia seeds
- ½ tsp. ground cinnamon
- ½ tsp. ground ginger
- ¼ tsp. ground cardamom
- ¼ tsp. ground cloves

Directions

1. In a small pan, heat the rice milk to just steaming. Steep the tea bags for 5 minutes, then discard.
2. In a blender, combine the rice milk, vanilla, ice, honey, chia seeds, cinnamon, ginger, cardamom, and cloves. Process until smooth, and serve.

Nutrition tip: To make this ahead, complete Step 1 and refrigerate the milk tea in an airtight container. When ready to make the smoothie, proceed as directed, reducing the ice to ½ c., and adding ¼ c. of water.

Nutrition

- Calories: 143
- Total fat: 5 g.
- Saturated fat: 1 g.
- Cholesterol: 0 mg.
- Carbohydrates: 19 g.
- Fiber: 6 g.
- Protein: 3 g.
- Phosphorus: 3 mg.
- Potassium: 93 mg.
- Sodium: 73 mg.

10.18   BERRY MINT WATER

Preparation time: 5 minutes - Cooking time: 0 minute - Servings: 8

Ingredients

- 8 c. water
- ½ c. strawberries
- ½ c. blackberries
- 3 mint sprigs

Directions

1. In a large pitcher, mix the water, strawberries, blackberries, and mint.
2. Cover and chill for at least 1 hour before drinking.
3. Store in the refrigerator for up to 2 days.

Nutrition tip: Substitute any of your favorite fruits in this recipe to create your own flavored water. You can also try out different herbs to add bold and complementary flavors. Some additional herbs that taste nice paired with fruit include cilantro, basil, rosemary, and thyme. Ginger root is another favorite water flavor enhancer that stimulates digestion and cleanses the kidneys.

Nutrition

- Calories: 7
- Total fat: 0 g.
- Saturated fat: 0 g.
- Cholesterol: 0 mg.
- Carbohydrates: 2 g.

- Fiber: 1 g.
- Protein: 0 g.
- Phosphorus: 4 mg.
- Potassium: 28 mg.
- Sodium: 0 mg.

10.19   HOMEMADE RICE MILK

Preparation time: 5 minutes - Cooking time: 0 minute - Servings: 4

Ingredients

- 1 c. long-grain white rice
- 4 c. water

- ½ tsp. vanilla extract (optional)

Directions

1. In a dry skillet, set at medium heat, toast the rice until lightly browned, about 5 minutes.
2. Transfer the rice to a jar or bowl, and add the water. Cover, refrigerate, and soak overnight.
3. In a blender, add the rice and water, along with the vanilla (if using), and process until smooth.
4. Place a fine-mesh strainer over a glass jar or bowl, and pour the milk into it. Serve immediately, or cover, refrigerate and serve within 3 days. Shake before using it.

Nutrition tip: Rice milk can be substituted in most recipes calling for whole milk or another nut milk as a low-fat, low-phosphorus, and low-potassium alternative. Use an equal amount of rice milk in place of other milk products, and proceed as directed in the recipe.

Nutrition

- Calories: 112
- Total fat: 0 g.
- Saturated fat: 0 g.
- Cholesterol: 0 mg.
- Carbohydrates: 24 g.
- Sodium: 80 mg.

- Fiber: 0 g.
- Protein: 0 g.
- Phosphorus: 0 mg.
- Potassium: 55 mg.

10.20   GINGER AND LEMON GREEN ICED-TEA

Preparation time: 5 minutes - Cooking time: 0 minute - Servings: 2

Ingredients

- 2 c. concentrated green or matcha tea, served hot
- 1 lemon, cut into wedges
- ¼ c. crystallized ginger, chopped into fine pieces

Directions

1. Get a glass container and mix the tea with the ginger and then cover and chill for 3 hours.
2. Strain and pour into serving glasses on top of ice if you wish.
3. Garnish with a wedge of lemon to serve.

Nutrition

- Calories: 20
- Fat: 0 g.
- Carbohydrates: 5 g.
- Phosphorus: 9 mg.
- Potassium: 106 mg.
- Sodium: 4 mg.
- Protein: 1 g.

CHAPTER 11 - CONCLUSION

You likely had little knowledge about your kidneys before. You probably did not know how you could take steps to improve your kidney health and decrease the risk of developing kidney failure. However, through reading this book, you now understand the power of the human kidney, as well as the prognosis of chronic kidney disease. While over 30 million Americans are being affected by kidney disease, you can now take steps to be one of the people who is actively working to promote your kidney health. Kidney disease now ranks as the 18th deadliest condition in the world.

These recipes are ideal whether you have been diagnosed with a kidney problem or you want to prevent any kidney issue.

With regards to your wellbeing and health, it is a smart thought to see your doctor as frequently as can to ensure you do not run into preventable issues that you need not get. The kidneys are your body's toxin channel (just like the liver), cleaning the blood of remote substances and toxins that are discharged from things like preservatives in the food and other toxins. When you eat flippantly and fill your body with toxins, either from nourishment, drinks (liquor or alcohol for instance), or even from the air you inhale (free radicals are in the sun and move through your skin, through messy air, and numerous food sources contain them). Your body additionally will in general convert numerous foods that appear to be benign until your body's organs convert them into chemicals like formaldehyde because of a synthetic response and transforming phase.

One case of this is a large portion of those diet sugars used in diet soft drinks, for instance, aspartame transforms into formaldehyde in the body. These toxins must be expelled, or they can prompt ailment, renal (kidney) failure, malignant growth, and various other painful problems.

This is not a condition that occurs without any forethought; it is a dynamic issue. It very well may be both found early and treated, diet changed, and fixed what is causing the issue. It is conceivable to have partial renal failure yet, as a rule; it requires some time (or downright awful diet for a short time) to arrive at absolute renal failure. You would prefer not to reach total renal failure since this will require standard dialysis treatments to save your life.

Dialysis treatments explicitly clean the blood of waste and toxins in the blood utilizing a machine in light of the fact that your body can no longer carry out the responsibility. Without treatments, you could die a very painful death. Renal failure can be the consequence of long-haul diabetes, hypertension, unreliable diet, and can stem from other health concerns.

A renal diet is tied in with directing the intake of protein and phosphorus in your eating routine. Restricting your sodium intake is likewise significant. By monitoring these 2 variables you can control the vast majority of the toxins/waste made by your body. This enables your kidney to a 100% correct functioning. In the event that you get a diagnosis early enough and truly moderate your diets with extraordinary consideration, you could avert all-out renal failure. In the event that you get this diet early, you can take out the issue completely.

CPSIA information can be obtained
at www.ICGtesting.com
Printed in the USA
BVHW052313040621
608823BV00007B/1126